PAINED

# PAINED

Uncomfortable Conversations about ·
the Public's Health

Michael D. Stein

AND

Sandro Galea

OXFORD
UNIVERSITY PRESS

# OXFORD
UNIVERSITY PRESS

Oxford University Press is a department of the University of Oxford. It furthers
the University's objective of excellence in research, scholarship, and education
by publishing worldwide. Oxford is a registered trade mark of Oxford University
Press in the UK and certain other countries.

Published in the United States of America by Oxford University Press
198 Madison Avenue, New York, NY 10016, United States of America.

Library of Congress Cataloging-in-Publication Data
Names: Stein, Michael D., 1960- author. | Galea, Sandro, author.
Title: Pained : uncomfortable conversations about the public's health /
Michael D. Stein, Sandro Galea.
Other titles: Uncomfortable conversations about the public's health
Description: New York : Oxford University Press, [2020] |
Includes bibliographical references and index.
Identifiers: LCCN 2019048246 (print) | LCCN 2019048247 (ebook) |
ISBN 9780197510384 (paperback) |
ISBN 9780197510407 (epub) | ISBN 9780197510414 (online)
Subjects: MESH: Social Determinants of Health | Public Health Practice |
Health Status Disparities | Socioeconomic Factors |
Attitude to Health | United States
Classification: LCC RA563.M56 (print) | LCC RA563.M56 (ebook) |
NLM WA 30 | DDC 362.1089—dc23
LC record available at https://lccn.loc.gov/2019048246
LC ebook record available at https://lccn.loc.gov/2019048247

1 3 5 7 9 8 6 4 2

Printed by Marquis, Canada

*This book is dedicated to Tobias Stein, Alexander Stein, and Hester Kaplan (MS), and to Isabel Tess Galea, Oliver Luke Galea, and Dr Margaret Kruk (SG).*

# CONTENTS

CONTENTS

## SECTION 2
# THE PERSONAL IS POLITICAL

## SECTION 3
# COUNTERINTUITIVE

CONTENTS

# SECTION 4
# A SURE ARGUMENT

# SECTION 5
# FOLLOW THE MONEY

CONTENTS

# SECTION 6
## DARK THOUGHTS

# SECTION 7
## THE FUNDAMENTALS

## SECTION 8
# WILL TECHNOLOGY SAVE US?

## SECTION 9
# WHAT NOBODY WANTS TO TALK ABOUT

# SECTION 10
# MAKING THINGS BETTER

When he was 21 years old, Benjamin Franklin gathered a select group of friends and neighbors—shoemakers, glass workers, students, surveyors—to create a weekly conversation circle he called the Junto Club. For the next 38 years, the Junto Club discussed the issues of the day and served as an incubator for many institutions in the public life of the 1700s which continue in American life today, including a lending library, a fire company, even a university. Franklin provided his group with a set of questions to guide each week's conversation.

In *Pained*, we gather 50 short essays and 20 data bytes that we hope will generate questions and stimulate conversation about health. We are, as a country, at a propitious time in our health conversation. We currently are in the middle of conversations that aim to push beyond the Affordable Care Act, Medicare for All, and the right to health care. These conversations, we argue, represent only a small portion of what the national conversation about health should be. We suggest here a wider list that includes a consideration of the forces that generate health and that goes beyond a focus on illness. While the book is explicitly political, it is in no way partisan—we aim to delight and incite readers of all political stripes.

As Franklin did, we ask questions in the service of inquiry; few of these essays offer answers. Not every essay imposes a necessity for great change, but we hope that each one engages its readers with questions about action, intention, and assumption.

By "Pained" we mean that these topics—from equity to poverty, from substance use to pollution—can be difficult, indeed uncomfortable, to discuss because they affect us on a visceral level: our bodies, our lives are at risk. While the book aims to capitalize on the preoccupations of this current heated political moment to take up new approaches to these topics of the day, it aspires to stand the test of time through robust, evidence-supported pieces that will interest readers, both general audience and expert, long into the future.

We think of these pieces as starters, talking points for topics that should be part of a citizen's foundation when discussing health. We intersperse surveys, tables, and graphs to enliven the text. The subjects we have chosen are meant to be an early alert system for what we believe really matters to the future health of the country, which we ignore at our peril. We hope these essays kick-start many new Junto Clubs.

# ACKNOWLEDGMENTS

We are indebted to many who have contributed to this book. This book emerged from a series of perspective pieces we published under the label "The Public's Health." That project was part of our ongoing Public Health Post (PHP) work at the Boston University School of Public Health. Melissa Davenport served as Managing Editor of PHP for its first two years, helping us create a vibrant new web site. Nick Diamond took over as Managing Editor and continued the tradition of excellence. PHP exists thanks to the original groundwork laid by Catherine Ettman, the early leadership of Professor David Jones, who served as its first Editor-in-Chief, and the Fellows who contribute to it daily. We are grateful to all. The databytes presented here were written originally by Fellows working under the editorial direction of Professor Jennifer Beard. In particular, thanks to Oluwatobi Alliyu, Gilbert Benavidez, Madeline Bishop, Jori Fortson, Julia Garcia, Greg Kantor, Chrissy Packtor, Erin Polka, Sampada Nandyala, and Qing Wai Wong. And last, but most definitely not least, this book would not be possible without the outstanding editorial assistance of Eric DelGizzo, who brought to the book, as he does to all our projects together, care, dedication, and facility with language that elevates all we do. Thank you.

# THINKING DIFFERENTLY

*Our health lags behind our peer countries, and a full consideration of health will require an engagement with issues that extend well beyond our medical systems. Fundamentally, health is much more than health care, and our health depends on much more than medicine.*

# [ 1 ]

# CREATING HEALTH IS LIKE WINNING AT SOCCER

Soccer is a global sport, played regularly by hundreds of millions of people. The game is simple: 11 players on one side try to get the ball into the net on the other side. Of the 11 players, only the goalie can use her hands to keep the ball from getting into the net.

Newcomers to soccer may, reasonably enough, see the goalie as the key to winning. After all, the goalie is the last defense, standing between the ball and the net. In theory, a spectacular goalie should be able to stop every shot that comes her way.

But anyone watching a professional soccer game will soon notice that the goalie spends most of the game prowling the space in front of her net, exhorting the other players to keep the ball away. Why? Well, a good goalie knows that no matter how good she is, she will not be able to keep certain balls out of the net. She knows the team will lose if there are too many shots on goal. Hence it is up to the other 10 players to keep the ball upfield, to make sure their team wins the game.

Soccer is a perfect metaphor for how societies can generate health. Health is shaped by the world around us—by the water we drink, by the air we breathe, by whether we live in a safe environment where exercise opportunities and healthy food are available to us, and by social policies that create a world free from inequity.

*Pained.* Michael D. Stein and Sandro Galea, Oxford University Press (2020). © Oxford University Press.
DOI: 10.1093/oso/9780197510384.001.0001

Imagine these conditions as the 10 soccer players moving the ball upfield, to maximize our chance of winning, of staying healthy.

## WHAT ABOUT THE GOALIE?

The goalie is medicine. It is our last resort—what can restore us to health if we get sick. We obviously want to have a very good goalie, a very good doctor, because we know that, every once in a while, there will be a shot on goal no matter how good the other 10 players are. But we also know that if we rely only on medicine we will not be healthy; we will simply be confronting disease after disease, until we lose.

We need a shift in the way we think about health. As in soccer, ten elevenths of our effort should be preventive, with medicine being our last line of defense. Health is about medicine, yes, but it is far more about the politics that create the world around us; about housing, transportation, and a livable wage; about community networks. Medicine is a small part of a larger "team" of forces that shape health.

## REFERENCE

265 million playing football. Fédération Internationale de Football Association Web Site. https://www.fifa.com/mm/document/fifafacts/bcoffsurv/emaga_9384_10704.pdf Published July 2007. Accessed September 10, 2019.

# [ 2 ]

# THE ILLUSION
# OF CLINICAL SUCCESS

As doctors, we have our fair share of patient success stories. A patient presents herself to our office or emergency room with a problem, we diagnose it, prescribe treatment, and the patient gets better. We can remember Lois, who presented with vomiting, whom we diagnosed with gastroenteritis, treated, and restored to health 2 weeks later. And Emmanuel, who came to the emergency department with a cut on his forehead because he fell down the stairs. He was sutured up, and the cut healed nicely. All clinicians have these stories. They are the reason why many of us went to medical school: to heal people, to make them better.

And yet anyone who has worked as a clinician knows what often happens next. The patient who had gastroenteritis returns again a few months later, this time with shortness of breath that turns out to be influenza pneumonia. The patient who had the cut on his forehead returns, this time with hepatitis. The reason for this, of course, is that these health issues had root causes that were not dealt with when we, the physicians, addressed the presenting complaint. Yes, the immediate concern was gastroenteritis, but the root cause was a refrigerator that went out when the electric bill was not paid, resulting in contaminated food. That same root cause—poor living conditions—resulted in the patient

*Pained.* Michael D. Stein and Sandro Galea, Oxford University Press (2020). © Oxford University Press.
DOI: 10.1093/oso/9780197510384.001.0001

catching pneumonia from an unvaccinated resident of his densely populated house. For the patient who presented with a fall and a cut, and later hepatitis, his medical problems were all related to alcohol dependence that had its roots in adolescence.

These observations are all immediately recognizable to clinicians who struggle to identify and treat illnesses whose sources often lie outside the medical system. That is what makes root causes so powerful: they escape ready treatment and underlie a multiplicity of medical presentations. The same root cause can be responsible for a gastrointestinal or a respiratory problem, for an injury or a hepatic problem. This is why, when we think of the causes of medical problems strictly from an organ-based perspective, it is never enough. Because medical problems often do not arise in their end organs; they are bodily manifestations of underlying issues.

These issues—such as inadequate housing, limited access to addiction treatment, poverty, and terrible neighborhoods—are *medical challenges*. What does this mean for the role of the clinician? Clinicians remain responsible for solving the immediate problem—the disease in front of them—but they must also grapple with the underlying causes. They can choose to become advocates, voices for public health outside of the hospital or clinic, or they can work within their day-to-day system, encouraging their hospital or clinic to embrace improving the underlying conditions that shape the health of patients. Absent this engagement, our clinical success remains fleeting, illusory.

# [ 3 ]

# CAN WE REVERSE COURSE ON HEALTH?

When it comes to promoting health, the United States lags behind all our high-income peer countries. Most well-informed readers know this; they know, for example, that we have lower life expectancy and higher mortality on multiple causes than Greece, France, or Norway—to name just a few of the nations currently ahead of us on health. Our health was not always this poor compared to other countries; as recently as the mid-1980s we were roughly in the middle of the pack of high-income nations, and we have since slowly fallen behind. And not just behind other high-income nations; we are also playing catch-up with less economically comparable countries, like Chile, Cuba, and Singapore.

One would think that, since we fell behind on health in a few decades—a blink of an eye in historical terms—we can reverse course and use the next few decades to catch up.

But can we? A 2018 paper published in the *American Journal of Public Health* suggests we cannot. The analysis found that, to achieve United Nations projected mortality estimates for Western Europe by 2030, US life expectancy must grow at 0.32% per year between now and then. Fewer than 10% of US states see health improving at that pace or higher; this makes it highly unlikely

*Pained.* Michael D. Stein and Sandro Galea, Oxford University Press (2020). © Oxford University Press.
DOI: 10.1093/oso/9780197510384.001.0001

that we are going to catch up. It suggests, in fact, we will fall further behind.

## WHY? THREE REASONS

First, in the United States, many gains in health and survival over the first half of the 20th century slowed significantly in the latter half of the last century and the first two decades of this one.

Second, we only excel at extending life for persons over 75. In this age group, we have lower mortality than other high-income countries. But even these gains appear to be diminishing, as we reach the natural limits of the human lifespan.

Third, we ignore the foundational forces that shape health. Data clearly show we persistently underinvest in education, efforts to promote healthy living, preventive care, and other programs and policies that address the root causes of health. Instead, we spend our money on inefficient and expensive health services.

It is odd that we should accept this state of affairs. Why does the United States spend more on health than any other country, but get less out of our spending than our peers? Shouldn't this be something that we talk about at every dinner table around the country until we change course? Food for thought indeed.

## REFERENCES

Galea S. *Well: what we need to talk about when we talk about health*. New York, NY: Oxford University Press; 2019.

Johnson C. The US spends more on health care than any other country. Here's what we're buying. *The Washington Post*. December 27, 2016. https://www.washingtonpost.com/news/wonk/wp/2016/12/27/

the-u-s-spends-more-on-health-care-than-any-other-country-heres-what-were-buying/ Accessed September 10, 2019.

Kindig D, Nobles J, Zidan M. Meeting the Institute of Medicine's 2030 US Life Expectancy Target. *American Journal of Public Health.* 2018; 108(1): 87–92. doi: 10.2105/AJPH.2017.304099

# [ 4 ]

# A PARTY TRICK

Here's a game you can play. At your next dinner party or discussion with friends, start a conversation about how to make Americans healthier. You can talk about anything you wish: the fact that health in America is getting worse, that the opioid epidemic has led to a life expectancy decline, or that firearms are a health problem. When you begin the conversation, start a timer in your head. Then see how long it takes for someone to use the word "health care" interchangeably with health.

Having played this game many times, we are confident in saying that this verbal swap will occur within 5 minutes. It rarely takes longer for someone to inadvertently say "health care" when she means "health."

Health and health care are very different things. Health is a desired state of well-being that allows us to do what we want to do, enabling us to live full, rich lives, and to realize our human potential. Health care is the system that aims to restore us to health when we get sick.

The conflation of health and health care is not without consequence. In fact, it fundamentally affects the health of our country. When we believe that health and health care are synonymous, we pour money into health care, thinking we are investing in health. This leads us away from addressing the true foundations of health,

*Pained*. Michael D. Stein and Sandro Galea, Oxford University Press (2020). © Oxford University Press.
DOI: 10.1093/oso/9780197510384.001.0001

such as early childhood education, parks and recreation, prevention of suicide and substance use, gender equity, and economic fairness. This results in a one-sided focus on health care, at the expense of investing in the roots causes of health.

Yet for all our investment in health care, our focus on doctors and medicine is not improving our health. We should be focusing on staying healthy to begin with, rather than on curing ourselves once we are already sick. We should change what we talk about when we discuss health, focusing on the root causes of health and disease, one conversation, one dinner party at a time.

# [ 5 ]

# TREATING LAURA

Laura is 42 years old. She is about 40 pounds overweight and has progressively worsening and painful osteoarthritis in her left knee. She has asthma, which keeps her out of work at least one day a month.

Laura's health issues would not be unusual to any primary care physician. When she goes to the doctor, he prescribes inhaled steroids for her asthma, anti-inflammatories for her arthritis, and recommends weight loss through better diet and exercise. Later, he guides Laura through the process of getting a knee replacement.

There is nothing wrong with this course of treatment. It is good care delivered by a responsible clinician. It is also comprehensive, addressing all of Laura's conditions. But it overlooks one key question: why did Laura get sick in the first place? Why is Laura, at a relatively young age, overweight, asthmatic, and in need of a knee replacement? How did all of this happen?

The answers lie in the circumstances of Laura's life. As the child of a single mother who had to work multiple jobs to keep the family afloat, Laura was raised eating the unhealthy processed food that was the only fare her mother could afford. This led to her becoming overweight at a young age. Her knee arthritis, a direct result of her weight, was compounded by her sedentary office job. Her asthma came from living in her childhood neighborhood,

*Pained.* Michael D. Stein and Sandro Galea, Oxford University Press (2020). © Oxford University Press.
DOI: 10.1093/oso/9780197510384.001.0001

where a pollution-spewing bus depot inflamed her airways and undermined her health.

So, while Laura needs treatment in the present, her medical conditions are a product of her past, of the world in which she grew up. Her physician can say to Laura that she should eat better and exercise more to lose weight, but how can she truly improve her health, when the best medicine would be for her to live her four decades over again, under healthier circumstances?

Laura was not well served by life's lottery. Some of us were luckier than she was in our circumstances of birth, some of us not. Critically, though, it is true for all of us that our health today is a product of our past and the conditions of our upbringing. If we could choose one thing to do to maximize our health, it would be to be born to high-income, well-educated parents who live in good neighborhoods, with access to all the resources that create health. Laura's doctor cannot give her these resources; only we can do that, by making a collective choice to build a world that generates health. We can keep treating Laura, and keep spending more and more money on health care, but until we invest in a world that produces, promotes, and supports health, we will always play catch-up. We can, and should, do better.

# [ 6 ]

# WATER QUALITY VIOLATIONS

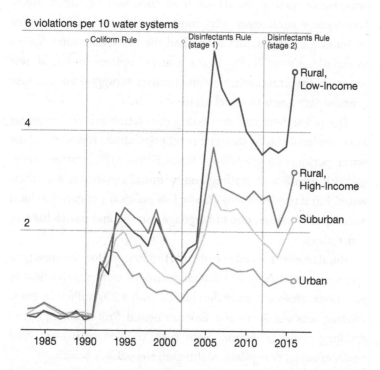

6 violations per 10 water systems

Most Americans have access to safe drinking water. But most isn't all. When we narrow our focus, we find that pockets of American communities are afflicted with high levels of contaminated water. While the country was focused on Flint, Michigan's lead in the water crisis in 2015, almost 10% of Americans were

*Pained.* Michael D. Stein and Sandro Galea, Oxford University Press (2020). © Oxford University Press.
DOI: 10.1093/oso/9780197510384.001.0001

drinking contaminated water that violated water quality standards. That's nearly 21 million people. Researchers at the University of California, Irvine, examined water quality violations across the United States from 1982 to 2015. They analyzed geographic and temporal patterns, with the goal of helping state enforcement agencies focus their attention on areas at high risk of contamination.

As depicted in the graph, rural areas were likelier to experience water quality violations than suburban or urban areas. Low-income rural areas were most affected, and rural counties of Texas, Oklahoma, and Idaho had the most violations. Spikes in violations were likelier to occur after implementation of new water quality standards, as communities struggled to decrease contaminant levels to match these standards.

The researchers cite decreasing population size and incomes as common obstacles faced by rural populations trying to follow water purification guidelines. Rural municipalities often struggle with insufficient staffing and technical capacity to test their water. Rural residents may also be less politically engaged in local water quality issues, due to language barriers and health literacy constraints.

Rural towns often rely on outside funding and low-interest government loans to support infrastructure to correct water quality violations. However, as of June 2017, over $600 million in grant funding was cut from the Environmental Protection Agency's drinking water programs. Such cuts, coupled with attempted environmental deregulation, threaten the public's health.

# REFERENCES

Allaire M, Wu H, Lall U. National trends in drinking water quality violations. *Proceedings of the National Academy of Sciences of the United States of America*. 2018; 115(9): 2078–83. doi: 10.1073/pnas.1719805115

Figure by David Gaitsgory, using data directly from the SDWIS Fed Reporting Services System.

Horn M. 26 Environmental rules being rolled back in the Trump era. Bloomberg Law Web site. https://www.bloomberglaw.com/document/ X28AOJ9S000000?bna_news_filter=environment-and-energy&jcsear ch=BNA%25200000016480c3d67aa7ec84f3ee1a0002#jcite Published July 12, 2018. Accessed September 11, 2019.

Safe Water Alliance, Environmental Justice Coalition for Water, International Human Rights Law Clinic, University of California, Berkeley, School of Law. Barriers to access to safe and affordable water for disadvantaged communities in California. https://www.law.berkeley.edu/wp-content/ uploads/2015/04/Shadow-Report-on-Right-to-Water-JS25-150511.pdf Accessed September 11, 2019.

USDA Provides $314 Million in Water and Waste Infrastructure Improvements in Rural Communities Nationwide. US Department of Agriculture Web site. https://www.usda.gov/media/press-releases/2015/11/02/ usda-provides-314-million-water-and-waste-infrastructure Accessed September 11, 2019.

Williams R. Study: Low income, rural areas most vulnerable to drinking water violations. Michigan Radio Web site. https://www.michiganradio.org/ post/study-low-income-rural-areas-most-vulnerable-drinking-water-violations Published February 20, 2018. Accessed September 11, 2019.

Wu M. How Trump's budget drains drinking water protections. Natural Resources Defense Council Web site. https://www.nrdc.org/experts/ how-trumps-budget-drains-drinking-water-protections Published June 19, 2017. Accessed September 11, 2019.

# THE IMMIGRANT EXPERIENCE
# IN HURRICANE SEASON

**Half of Immigrants with Home Damage Said They Worried
Seeking Help Would Draw Attention to Legal Status**

AMONG TEXAS GULF COAST RESIDENTS WHO HAD ANY DAMAGE TO THEIR HOME AS A RESULT OF HURRICANE HARVEY: How worried are you, if at all, that if you try to get help in recovering from Hurricane Harvey, you will draw attention to your or a family member's immigration status?

■ Very worried ■ Somewhat worried ■ Not too worried ▢ Not at all worried

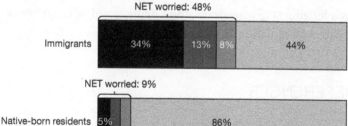

NOTE: Don't know/Refused responses not shown.
SOURCE: KFF/EHF *Texas Post-Heavy Survey* (conducted Oct. 17-Nov. 20, 2017)

In August of 2017, Hurricane Harvey ravaged Texas, threatening the health and safety of Gulf Coast residents. The effects of the storm were especially painful for immigrant families, many of whom feared that reporting property damage and losses caused by Harvey would draw negative attention from governmental

*Pained.* Michael D. Stein and Sandro Galea, Oxford University Press (2020). © Oxford University Press.
DOI: 10.1093/oso/9780197510384.001.0001

authorities. These fears were heightened by the actions of Border Patrol, who kept checkpoints open immediately after the storm.

The Kaiser Family Foundation published survey findings on the impact of Harvey on immigrants living along the Texas Gulf Coast. The figure shows that immigrants with homes hit by Harvey reported feeling more worried about seeking help for storm-related damages than their native-born counterparts. About 34% of immigrants responded that they were very worried that reaching out for help would highlight their own or a family member's status. Only 5% of native-born residents responded similarly. Immigrants were also less likely to have flood or home insurance, or to apply for governmental disaster assistance. Notably, the Federal Emergency Management Agency's policies do not guarantee Disaster Unemployment Assistance to undocumented individuals. For these reasons, fear of disclosing immigration status may act as a barrier to immigrants seeking help and to broader efforts to ameliorate storm damage and safeguard health in the wake of natural disasters.

# REFERENCES

Figure from Wu B, Hamel L, Brodie M, Sim S, Marks E. Hurricane Harvey: The experiences of immigrants living in the Texas Gulf Coast. Kaiser Family Foundation Web site. https://www.kff.org/disparities-policy/report/hurricane-harvey-experiences-immigrants-texas-gulf-coast/ Published March 20, 2018. Accessed September 11, 2019.

Questions and Answers for Undocumented Immigrants Regarding FEMA Assistance. Federal Emergency Management Agency Web site. https://www.fema.gov/news-release/2004/06/17/questions-and-answers-undocumented-immigrants-regarding-fema-assistance Accessed September 11, 2019.

Romero S, Jordan M. It was an uneasy time for immigrants in Texas. Then the rains came. *The New York Times*. August 29, 2017. https://www.nytimes.com/2017/08/29/us/immigration-harvey-border-patrol.html Accessed September 11, 2019.

# THE PERSONAL IS POLITICAL

*The national political conversation matters to our health. Climate change, the census, community policing, and political rhetoric all shape how healthy we, as citizens, are able to be. What do we need to know about the politics of these issues to inform a better conversation about health?*

# [ 8 ]

# DENYING CLIMATE CHANGE IS DENYING HEALTH

In recent years, global environmental climate change has become a third rail in American culture, dividing us along political lines. The Republican party espouses a range of positions, from the denial of climate change (i.e., the earth is not getting warmer) to denial of our role in causing the problem (i.e., even if climate change exists, humans have nothing to do with it). Each of these positions amounts to inaction on climate change. The Democratic Party falls more in line with the science on this issue, which is largely settled. There is little disagreement among scientists that the earth is getting warmer. Hence, the political argument is not really about the science as much as it is about priorities. The Republican Party—in the past several decades a ceaselessly pro-market party—prioritizes deregulation and corporate interests over the potential disruption of these interests caused by the structural changes necessary to address climate change. The Democratic Party, for its part, has increasingly chosen to prioritize the future of the planet over the unfettered primacy of markets.

Climate change happens slowly; its worst consequences may not affect us for generations to come. How, then, do we make the decision to take the politically difficult steps today to protect our world tomorrow?

*Pained*. Michael D. Stein and Sandro Galea, Oxford University Press (2020). © Oxford University Press.
DOI: 10.1093/oso/9780197510384.001.0001

This is where health can inform the conversation. We all value health. Our national health care spending is a testament to how much we are willing to invest in staying healthy. And make no mistake: climate change threatens health. The World Health Organization (WHO) estimates that between 2030 and 2050, climate change is expected to cause approximately 250,000 additional deaths per year, from malnutrition, malaria, diarrhea, and heat stress. A 2018 paper shows that unmitigated climate change will result in up to 40,000 additional suicides across the United States and Mexico by 2050. In two decades, as a direct result of climate change, the number of natural disasters doubled from approximately 200 to 400 per year, with human costs rising commensurately. The 2017 hurricane season far exceeded any season in the preceding 30 years. The list goes on.

When we recognize that climate change matters for health, we open the door for health to become an organizing principle in addressing this issue. If we do not act on climate change, we are compromising our health. Perhaps we are fine with that. More likely, though, the vast majority of us are not fine with it, and if we properly weigh the impact of climate change on our health today and in the years to come, the politics of this issue would be very different.

## REFERENCES

AR5 Synthesis Report: Climate Change 2014. Intergovernmental Panel on Climate Change Web site. http://www.ipcc.ch/report/ar5/syr/ Accessed September 11, 2019.

Burke M, González F, Baylis P, et al. Higher temperatures increase suicide rates in the United States and Mexico. *Nature Climate Change*. 2018; 8: 723–29.

Climate change and health. World Health Organization Web site. https://www.who.int/news-room/fact-sheets/detail/climate-change-and-health Published February 1, 2018. Accessed September 11, 2019.

Climate change, natural disasters and human displacement: a UNHCR perspective. United Nations High Commissioner for Refugees Web site. https://www.unhcr.org/4901e81a4.html Accessed September 11, 2019.

Pierre-Louis K. Why is the cold weather so extreme if the earth is warming? *The New York Times*. January 31, 2019. https://www.nytimes.com/interactive/2019/climate/winter-cold-weather.html?mtrref=www.publichealthpost.org&assetType=REGIWALL Accessed September 11, 2019.

Stone M. Trump's NASA pick says human-caused climate change depends "on a whole lot of factors." November 1, 2017. *Gizmodo*. https://earther.gizmodo.com/trumps-nasa-pick-says-human-caused-climate-change-depen-1820043856 Accessed September 11, 2019.

# [ 9 ]

# PUBLIC HEALTH AND A PRESIDENT'S RACISM

In 2018, President Trump suggested that the United States should not be granting admission to people from what he referred to as "shithole" countries. He appeared to be talking about Haiti, El Salvador, and African nations with predominantly nonwhite populations. That a President of the United States used such terminology appropriately resulted in a collective furor. There seems little question that Trump's words fell far beneath the level of dignity and decorum one might expect from the leader of the United States. But why did the president's racism matter for the health of the public?

To answer this question, one needs to understand where health comes from. Health is the product of the social, economic, and cultural context in which we live. This context is also shaped by social norms that do much to determine our behaviors and their consequences. Changing these norms can produce both positive and negative health effects.

On the positive side, changing norms can promote health, by making unacceptable unhealthy conditions and behaviors that were once common, even celebrated. This was evident in the decline in cigarette smoking and motor vehicle deaths in the United States during the latter half of the 20th century; the

*Pained.* Michael D. Stein and Sandro Galea, Oxford University Press (2020). © Oxford University Press. DOI: 10.1093/oso/9780197510384.001.0001

former was attributable to change in public perceptions about smoking and the latter to a widespread acceptance of vehicular and road safety measures.

On the negative side, changing norms for the worse can empower elements of hate in society. The office of the president has the largest megaphone in the world. When a president promotes hate, it shifts norms, suggesting that hate *does* in fact have a place in our country and our world. This opens the door to more hate crimes, more exclusion of minority groups from salutary resources, and little to no effort to address racial health gaps.

Racism is morally repugnant. It needs no link to health to be considered unacceptable. Yet by making discrimination and cruelty mainstream, racist comments present a clear threat to the health of populations—especially when they are made by a president.

## REFERENCES

Embury-Dennis T. UN calls Donald Trump's s***hole immigrants comments "racist." *The Independent*. January 12, 2018. https://www.independent. co.uk/news/world/americas/un-donald-trump-shithole-immigrants-haiti-africa-racist-huamn-rights-united-nations-a8155186.html Accessed September 11, 2019.

Petulla S. The number of hate crimes rose in 2016. *CNN*. November 13, 2017. https://edition.cnn.com/2017/11/13/politics/hate-crimes-fbi-2016-rise/index.html Accessed September 11, 2019.

# THE CENSUS AND PUBLIC HEALTH

The US Constitution mandates that each resident of the country be counted at least every 10 years. As the 2020 census approached, the Trump administration launched an effort to meddle with how to perform this head count, by adding a question about citizenship to the census. This move was roundly criticized by the Census Bureau's Scientific Advisory committee and became the target of lawsuits. It looked very much like an attempt to depress the 2020 population count in immigrant-rich and predominantly Democratic areas, in advance of redistricting in 2021. Tying population data to law enforcement made some worry that as many as 24 million people would not participate and be counted—those who owe child support, for example, or who are behind on student loan payments—because they fear their names and addresses might be shared with police.

Accurate census data are critical for the public's health. These data drive federal grants to states for the Special Supplemental Nutrition Program for Women, Infants, and Children. They determine funding for Medicaid and for school lunch programs. They guide disaster response and disease outbreak planning. The Centers for Disease Control and Prevention (CDC) uses census information to locate geographic areas with low education levels

*Pained*. Michael D. Stein and Sandro Galea, Oxford University Press (2020). © Oxford University Press. DOI: 10.1093/oso/9780197510384.001.0001

and high poverty rates, so as to expand screening and outreach programs. These data inform the building of roads, schools, and health centers.

For these reasons, political moves to influence the census is a matter of great concern for public health. It is another example of why health is ultimately inseparable from the political landscape in which we live.

# REFERENCES

Prokop A. Trump's census citizenship question fiasco, explained. *Vox*. July 11, 2019. https://www.vox.com/2019/7/11/20689015/census-citizenship-question-trump-executive-order. Accessed September 11, 2019.

Shapiro R. Trump's Census policy could boomerang and hurt red states as well as blue states. Brookings Web site. https://www.brookings.edu/blog/fixgov/2018/03/30/trump-census-harms-red-blue-states/ Published March 30, 2018. Accessed September 11, 2019.

# [ 11 ]

# WHEN WE TALK ABOUT PUBLIC HEALTH

During the 2016 presidential campaign, there was little discussion by candidates Donald Trump and Hillary Clinton of public health issues.

A study that combed the texts of major campaign speeches, interviews, and advertisements made by candidates Trump and Clinton for public health keywords concluded, "the two candidates did not communicate the major concerns of the public health field." The study authors bemoaned that general references to "health" accounted for less than 1% of the words used by the candidates.

It is worth noting what the authors of the study considered to be "health topics." The study focused on six "public health issues": wellness, diet, disease prevention, substance abuse, workplace standards, and vaccinations.

We do not disagree that these are public health issues. We suggest, however, that it would be a shame if this short list constitutes our entire political discourse about public health.

Housing, health disparities, immigration, aging, mental health and substance use, military medicine, the environment, criminal justice, food policy, health technology, disability/injury,

*Pained.* Michael D. Stein and Sandro Galea, Oxford University Press (2020). © Oxford University Press.
DOI: 10.1093/oso/9780197510384.001.0001

and health care delivery—this is something closer to the full list of forces that shape the public's health in contemporary America.

We suspect that politicians and the public already use more than 1% of their words discussing these topics. Immigration and military issues, for example, have dominated the political debate in recent years. But the public health implications of these issues are rarely addressed. We talk about putting undocumented immigrants in detention centers, but what happens when we do not screen for and treat tuberculosis among these immigrants? We talk about military budgets, but we do not talk about the costs of posttraumatic stress disorder (PTSD)—only one of the many hidden health costs of war—to the single-payer insurance system that our military uses.

If there is a unifying theme left in our divided country, it is that we all want to be healthier. The goal of improving health should drive our policies and our political discourse. Every budget, every piece of policy, can and should be conceived with health in mind. We can do this, if we can only summon the political will.

## REFERENCE

Hatcher W, Vick A. Public health issues in 2016 presidential campaign communications. *American Journal of Public Health*. 2018; 108(2): 191–92. doi: 10.2105/AJPH.2017.304221

# [ 12 ]

# THE TWO-DEGREE SOLUTION

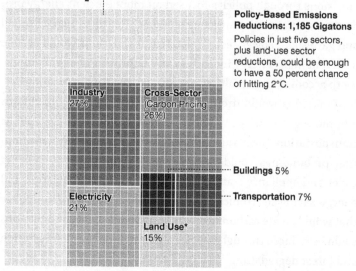

**Business As Usual Cumulative Emissions, 2020–2050:**
**2,253 Gigatons $CO_2$e**

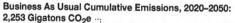

**Policy-Based Emissions**
**Reductions: 1,185 Gigatons**
Policies in just five sectors, plus land-use sector reductions, could be enough to have a 50 percent chance of hitting 2°C.

Industry
27%

Cross-Sector
(Carbon Pricing
26%)

···· **Buildings** 5%

Electricity
21%

···· **Transportation** 7%

Land Use*
15%

*Land-use emissions are calculated separately in this book, as explained in chapter two.*

Our globe is on a fast track to exceed 2°C in warming by 2050, which will inevitably lead to more extreme weather events. How can we avoid this scenario and its consequences for health? An energy policy firm, Energy Innovation, tackled that question by modeling how current energy policies would impact future emissions.

*Pained*. Michael D. Stein and Sandro Galea, Oxford University Press (2020). © Oxford University Press.
DOI: 10.1093/oso/9780197510384.001.0001

To have a 50% chance of not overshooting 2°C by 2050, we must reduce our carbon emissions by 1156 gigatons, or 41%, from what we might expect to produce over the next 30 years. This is achievable if the top 20 greenhouse gas–emitting countries (with China and the United States in the lead) reduce their emissions. The figure illustrates the cumulative emissions that need to (and can) be reduced across five sectors of the economy, and land use, in order to remain below the most dangerous levels in 2050.

Industry has the greatest potential for cutting back on global emissions through policies focused on more efficient energy production and stricter emissions standards (such as regulating oil and gas leaks). Power sector (electricity) emissions would decline with renewable energy incentives and improving the grid's capacity to accommodate multiple energy sources. Transportation sector emissions would drop with stricter fuel economy standards and more green urban transportation systems (improved public transportation, bike lanes, and sidewalks). The energy consumption of buildings could decrease with more efficient building codes and appliance standards (such as improved insulation and energy-saving electronics). Carbon pricing is a cross-sector policy that would create carbon taxes and caps, while land use emissions could be reduced through policies aimed at reducing deforestation and forest degradation.

The Paris Agreement provided targets for reducing emissions, but only policy implementation will allow us to meet them in time. We have access to clear guidelines for what we need to do to curb our emissions for a safer future. How to make the necessary changes is less clear, but it will certainly be impossible without focused and concerted international effort, and robust engagement with the politics of this issue.

# REFERENCES

Building codes and appliance standards. Energy Innovation Web site. https://www.energypolicy.solutions/policies/building-codes-appliance-standards/ Accessed September 12, 2019.

Carbon pricing. Energy Innovation Web site. https://www.energypolicy.solutions/policies/carbon-pricing/ Accessed September 12, 2019.

Complementary power sector policies. Energy Innovation Web site. https://www.energypolicy.solutions/policies/complementary-electricity-policies/ Accessed September 12, 2019.

Controlling industrial greenhouse gas emissions. Center for Climate and Energy Solutions Web site. https://www.c2es.org/content/regulating-industrial-sector-carbon-emissions/ Accessed September 12, 2019.

Do the math. Energy Innovation Web site. https://www.energypolicy.solutions/do-the-math/ Accessed September 12, 2019.

Energy Innovation Web site. https://energyinnovation.org Accessed September 12, 2019.

Figure from How to Prioritize Policies for Emissions Reduction. Energy Innovation Web site. https://www.energypolicy.solutions/how-to-prioritize-policies/ Accessed September 12, 2019.

Harvey H, Orvis R, Rissman J. *Designing climate solutions: a policy guide for low-carbon energy*. Washington, DC: Island Press; 2018.

Industrial energy efficiency. Energy Innovation Web site. https://www.energypolicy.solutions/policies/industrial-energy-efficiency/ Accessed September 12, 2019.

Industrial process emissions policies. Energy Innovation Web site. https://www.energypolicy.solutions/policies/industrial-process-emissions-policies/ Accessed September 12, 2019.

Policy design to win on climate. Energy Innovation Web site. https://www.energypolicy.solutions/guide/ Accessed September 12, 2019.

Renewable portfolio standards and feed-in tariffs. Energy Innovation Web site. https://www.energypolicy.solutions/policies/feed-in-tariffs/ Accessed September 12, 2019.

Urban mobility policies. Energy Innovation Web site. https://www.energypolicy.solutions/policies/urban-mobility-policies/ Accessed September 12, 2019.

Vehicle performance standards. Energy Innovation Web site. https://www.energypolicy.solutions/policies/vehicle-performance-standards/ Accessed September 12, 2019.

What are the best policies to solve climate change? Energy Innovation Web site. https://us.energypolicy.solutions Accessed September 12, 2019.

# [ 13 ]

# THE PARTISAN DIVIDE OVER
# A SODA TAX

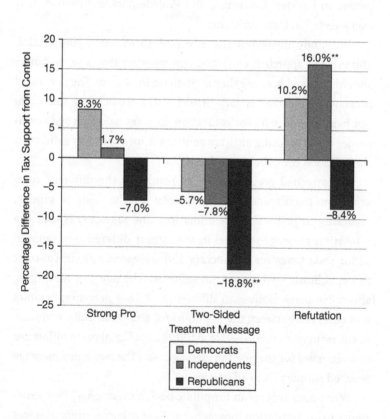

*Pained.* Michael D. Stein and Sandro Galea, Oxford University Press (2020). © Oxford University Press.
DOI: 10.1093/oso/9780197510384.001.0001

Public health messaging is arguably just as important as public health policies. Passing and implementing policies is often contingent on favorable public opinion.

Researchers Sarah Gollust, Colleen Barry, and Jeff Nierderdeppe examined messaging in the context of partisan responses to a public health initiative—a sugary drink tax. Many cities across the United States have proposed such a policy. The tax is controversial, facing opposition fueled and funded by the soda industry. As of this writing, the sugary drink tax has been passed in Berkley, California, and Philadelphia, Pennsylvania. It was rejected in New York City.

The study measured the effect of three messaging tactics. The pro-tax approach conveyed the message that sugary drinks should be taxed because they contribute to obesity. The two-sided message stated that sugary drinks cause obesity, but taxes will not help to reduce it. The refutation message said that soda companies are promoting anti-tax sentiment for their own gain, even though soda contributes to obesity.

The attached graph shows the results of the different messages on participants in comparison to the control groups, according to political party affiliation. The takeaway is that the refutation message resulted in the largest difference of opinion about soda taxes for Democrats and Independents, in contrast to Republicans—who were not influenced by negative messaging about company motives. A difference of 18.4 percentage points was observed between the Republicans' and Democrats' response to the refutation message. No significant political party difference was observed for the pro-tax message. And the two-sided message reduced support from all parties.

What does this mean for public health messaging? Past experience using refutation messaging against tobacco companies was quite successful in moving policymakers to pass tobacco taxes.

Current campaigns for a soda tax have begun to introduce rhetoric against soda companies. Messaging using "Big Soda" was the third most popular pro-tax argument in Richmond, El Monte, and Telluride, Colorado. If the study findings play out in real life, messages blaming soda companies for callous motives may be effective with Democrats and Independents but could alienate Republicans.

Failed attempts to implement a soda tax in many major US cities show just how ferocious opposition to such measures can be. Philadelphia was the first major US city to implement the tax. Instead of focusing on health benefits or "Big Soda," Mayor Jim Kenney pushed the tax as a much-needed source of revenue. Perhaps it is time to look outside the conventional arguments when policymakers attempt to pass soda taxes.

## REFERENCES

Bottemiller Evich H. Philly's soda tax may be turning point. *Politico*. June 16, 2016. https://www.politico.com/story/2016/06/soda-tax-philadelphia-224442 Accessed September 12, 2019.

Figure from Gollust SE, Barry CL, Niederdeppe J. Partisan responses to public health messages: motivated reasoning and sugary drink taxes. *Journal of Health Politics, Policy and Law*. 2017; 42(6): 1005–37. doi: 10.1215/03616878-4193606

Nixon L, Mejia P, Cheyne A, Dorfman L. Big Soda's long shadow: news coverage of local proposals to tax sugar-sweetened beverages in Richmond, El Monte and Telluride. *Critical Public Health*. 2015; 25(3): 333–47. doi: 10.1080/09581596.2014.987729

# COUNTERINTUITIVE

*Do we realize that more children are killed by guns in the United States than die of cancer? That when we try to improve population health, we often widen health gaps? That our national fascination with gut microbiota will likely do nothing for our health, even as it distracts us from what matters? The reality of what improves our health and what threatens it often goes against the grain of our assumptions.*

# WHAT KILLS OUR KIDS?

One of the greatest triumphs in health over the past century has been the dramatic decrease in childhood mortality. And yet children still die. Until this is no longer so, we should be looking carefully at what kills our children and asking what we can do about it.

In 2016, there were, in the United States, about 38,000 deaths of children under the age of 19. Roughly half of deaths occur in early childhood due to genetic conditions, chromosomal abnormalities, and other perinatal conditions, many of which we do not know how to treat. But most of the other half we should be able to prevent. The vast majority of these deaths are due to injury—a combination of car accidents, gun-related deaths, suffocation in early childhood, drowning, and drug overdose. The two leading causes of injury deaths are motor vehicle deaths (nearly 4,000) and gun-related deaths (nearly 3,000). Understanding how to prevent them can provide a template for stopping other childhood deaths.

When it comes to motor vehicle deaths, we are tackling the problem step by step. The Vision Zero initiative, passed by the Swedish parliament 20 years ago, aims to reduce traffic fatalities to zero. The effort—which includes monitoring traffic flow and vehicle technology solutions such as novel automatic braking systems—has dramatically reduced fatalities, not just for

*Pained.* Michael D. Stein and Sandro Galea, Oxford University Press (2020). © Oxford University Press. DOI: 10.1093/oso/9780197510384.001.0001

travelers in cars, but also for pedestrians whose fatality rate has decreased by more than 50%.

The Vision Zero initiative is predicated on a simple idea: "We are human and make mistakes." As such, we need to design safer roads and cars to keep us safe. Rather than aim for perfection—by trying, for example, to make people into ideal drivers—the initiative accepts us as we are and strives to create a world where we can be both fallibly human and healthy at the same time. Such an approach is at the heart of most effective prevention strategies.

We have yet to fully apply this approach to the other major cause of injury and death: guns. But just like motor vehicle accidents, childhood deaths from guns will not end until we work to create a safer environment by reducing the availability of firearms. Multiple low-tech firearm features can prevent accidental gun discharges, including heavier trigger pulls and grip safeties. No federal agency oversees how guns are designed or built, even though federal safety regulations are standard for other consumer products, like cars. More broadly, our spending on preventing injury, including gun injury, is abysmally low. System design takes human fallibility into account, and it can protect children. Let's spend some of our research dollars there.

## REFERENCES

Child health. Centers for Disease Control and Prevention Web site. https://www.cdc.gov/nchs/fastats/child-health.htm Accessed September 12, 2019.

Stark DE, Shah NH. Funding and publication of research on gun violence and other leading causes of death. *JAMA: The Journal of the American Medical Association.* 2017; 317(1): 84–85. doi: 10.1001/jama.2016.16215

Under-five mortality. United Nations Children's Fund Web site. https://data.unicef.org/topic/child-survival/under-five-mortality/ Published March 2018. Accessed September 12, 2019.

Vision Zero Network Web site. https://visionzeronetwork.org Accessed September 12, 2019.

Vision Zero: Learning from Sweden's successes. Center for Active Design Web site. https://centerforactivedesign.org/visionzero Accessed September 12, 2019.

# [ 15 ]

# WHAT DATA DO WE NEED FOR HEALTH?

We spend an inordinate amount of money on health care. Much of this spending goes to data acquisition, to medical monitoring, and to assessment of how our health systems function. But are there other areas where money devoted to gathering health data might be better spent?

Our health is a product of the world around us. This is perhaps most easily understood by thinking about how much time we spend in the various places where we live, work, and gather.

Data from the Bureau of Labor Statistics offer a picture of these places. Out of 8,736 hours in a year, we spend more than half, or about 4,566, at home. We spend 1,893 hours in our workplaces or 1,198 at school. We spend 93 hours in places of worship. Far down the list, at 15 hours a year, are interactions with the health care delivery system.

That picture is enough to make two things clear.

First, insofar as health is shaped by where and how we live, it is a product of where we are *between* visits to doctors and hospitals. We are simply not in contact with the health care system very often. It must be something, then, about all the time we spend away from medical care that determines our health.

*Pained.* Michael D. Stein and Sandro Galea, Oxford University Press (2020). © Oxford University Press. DOI: 10.1093/oso/9780197510384.001.0001

Second, because health care is really a small part of our life, it should not take up too much of our health improvement time or attention. Ultimately, medical care is a means to an end, and that end is living a full and satisfying life.

With this in mind, we revisit the question we started with: what data do we need to generate better health? We need data about how all that other "nonmedical" time that shapes our health.

The apps and systems that collect data should be used to gather information on home life, time spent at work, and time spent in schools and in places of worship—the time that truly shapes people's health. Innovation in this area of data collection could break new ground, paying dividends for those who pioneer it, and for those who reap the health benefits of these emerging tools.

## REFERENCE

American time use survey summary. Bureau of Labor Statistics Web site. https://www.bls.gov/news.release/atus.nr0.htm Accessed September 12, 2019.

# [ 16 ]

# WE CANNOT HAVE IT ALL

Imagine for a moment that you are the health commissioner responsible for a town of 100,000 people. The mayor calls you into her office and reminds you that one of her campaign promises was to improve the town's flu vaccination rate. The previous season, 45% of the town's residents received the vaccine. This season, the mayor wants the vaccination rate to hit 65%. That all sounds reasonable, and with your team you develop a strategy that communicates, primarily through doctors' offices, the importance of flu vaccinations. You develop written material and some videos, and you make sure that all patients see them prominently displayed. The strategy works. At the end of this year's flu season, you have vaccinated 65% of everyone in town.

But this success is not as complete as it looks. An analyst in the health department examines the data a bit more carefully. She notes that the town is divided into two groups. Half the town, in its wealthier north section, had a flu vaccination rate that was already 60% when you started. It rose to 90% at the end of the campaign. The southern, poorer half of town had a vaccination rate of 30% when you started; it rose to 40% by the end of the campaign. Therefore, you increased the vaccination rate by 30% among the rich, and by 10% among the poor, many of whom do not get to doctors' offices and, as such, did not benefit much from

*Pained*. Michael D. Stein and Sandro Galea, Oxford University Press (2020). © Oxford University Press.
DOI: 10.1093/oso/9780197510384.001.0001

your campaign. Your rich-poor gap in vaccination was 30% when you started; it was 50% when you finished.

So, did your campaign work?

At the level of what the mayor promised in her campaign—that more residents would be vaccinated—it did. In fact, you increased vaccination rates overall by 20%, which is no mean feat. And you can point to the fact that the rates of vaccination improved among everyone. Yes, they increased less in the poor parts of town, but they did increase.

But the health gaps in town between the rich and the poor residents also increased—substantially. This illustrates what economists call an equity/efficiency trade-off. In other words: we cannot have it all. As long as we design interventions that privilege populations that are already well-off, we will be widening the gaps between health haves and health have-nots, even if we improve overall health.

Recognizing that we cannot have it all, is this trade-off worth it? Answering this question comes down to our values. While improving overall health may create some impressive numbers, how satisfied should we be with this progress, when it comes at the expense of further marginalizing an already vulnerable group?

Health inequities like these are the result of systematic injustice—in this case, the injustice of unequal access to health care settings where vaccine marketing and delivery take place, and the broader socioeconomic inequality this reflects. These inequities matter. After all, if a pocket of the town's population remains unvaccinated, it puts the whole area at risk, even if vaccination rates go up among the rich. Public health must not allow lopsided interventions like these to occur. It must recognize that a healthy society is one where health is accessible to all—not some, or even most, but all.

# [ 17 ]

# THE MICROBIOME AND THE PUBLIC'S HEALTH

Each of us is a living ecosystem with trillions of microorganisms living on and in us—our microbiome. Each of us has her own collection of such microbes, inhabiting skin, mouth, gut, and lungs. Much about our microbiome is surprising. It is surprising that identical twins are barely more similar to one another in microbial composition than are nonidentical twins; that our personal menagerie changes over time; that a sufficiently extreme short-term dietary change can cause the gastrointestinal flora of different people to resemble one another within days.

The microbiome may well turn out to play a critical role in an individual's health, which is a very intriguing prospect. But when nearly two dozen federal agencies—NIH, FDA, EPA, and NSF—join together to release a five-year strategic plan to bolster the study of microbiomes, we wonder why these same agencies can't get together on another day to make a second strategic plan. This one would be a plan for public health, not private health, one that could save lives and reduce morbidities next year by focusing on what we *know* matters to our health, the policies that drive behavior.

We are at that moment in a relatively new scientific field when everything seems to influence it; the microbiome's composition is

*Pained*. Michael D. Stein and Sandro Galea, Oxford University Press (2020). © Oxford University Press.
DOI: 10.1093/oso/9780197510384.001.0001

altered by sleep, stress, and exercise. We, who work far from the basic science lab, believe it would indeed be meaningful if, someday, by controlling our behaviors, we might know how to control our personal microbial community and thus our health. Yet a "personalized" microbiome remains a distant and unlikely dream.

We agree with our microbiomist colleagues that our environment, from the personal to the atmospheric, matters. And that our social networks, with whom and how we interact, matter too. But we would prioritize attention to the *known* drivers of longevity and quality of life for today's population—such as poverty, insurance gaps, homelessness, the broad distribution of preventive services. These are hard problems that we can change, and which would benefit from strategic health planning. We are envious that the microbiome brought 23 federal agencies together in common cause, even if their report included the usual recommendations: share data, make access to data easier, collaborate, and expand the number of studies.

Let's appreciate microbiome research for what it is—pure, joyous, creative science that may produce fascinating new findings in a decade or two and in the meantime a workforce development venture for young scientists. But let's collaborate on equally hard macro-level puzzles that may better and sooner benefit the public's health.

## REFERENCES

Benedict C, Vogel H, Jonas W, et al. Gut microbiota and glucometabolic alterations in response to recurrent partial sleep deprivation in normal-weight young individuals. *Molecular Metabolism.* 2016; 5(12): 1175–86. doi: 10.1016/j.molmet.2016.10.003

Cook MD, Allen JM, Pence BD, et al. Exercise and gut immune function: Evidence of alterations in colon immune cell homeostasis and microbiome characteristics with exercise training. *Immunology & Cell Biology*. 2016; 94(2): 158–63. doi: 10.1038/icb.2015.108

David LA, Materna AC, Friedman J, et al. Host lifestyle affects human microbiota on daily timescales. *Genome Biology*. 2014; 15(7): R89.

Karl JP, Margolis LM, Madslien EH, et al. Changes in intestinal microbiota composition and metabolism coincide with increased intestinal permeability in young adults under prolonged physiological stress. *American Journal of Physiology: Gastrointestinal and Liver Physiology*. 2017; 312(6): G559–G571. doi: 10.1152/ajpgi.00066.2017

# [ 18 ]

# IMMIGRANTS AND PRIVATE INSURANCE

*Pay More, Use Less*

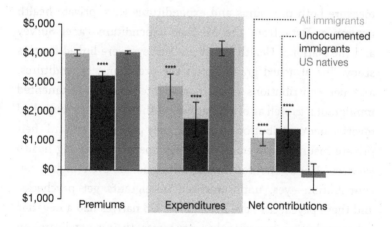

PER CAPITA PREMIUMS, ADJUSTED
EXPENDITURES, AND NET
CONTRIBUTIONS TO PRIVATE HEALTH
INSURANCE, BY NATIVITY STATUS, 2014

In the United States, it is not uncommon to hear that immigrants,
particularly undocumented immigrants, are labeled as a "drag" on

*Pained.* Michael D. Stein and Sandro Galea, Oxford University Press (2020). © Oxford University Press.
DOI: 10.1093/oso/9780197510384.001.0001

the system, a group that takes advantage of societal resources at the expense of native-born citizens. Leaving aside the moral question of whether any group is more or less entitled than any other to access the resources necessary to live a healthy life, how true is this accusation, in the context of health care? Do immigrants really use the system more, but pay less, at the "expense" of everyone else?

In fact, the opposite is true. Between 2002 and 2009, immigrants paid an estimated $115.2 billion more into Medicare than they used. And what of private insurance, which covers half of all immigrants in the United States? A 2018 *Health Affairs* study used data from the Medical Expenditure Panel Survey (MEPS) to measure both premiums and expenditures from private health insurance. Data from the Medical Expenditure Panel Survey and the National Health Interview Surveys were linked for this study. The attached graph shows the premiums, expenditures, and net contributions of all documented and undocumented immigrants, as well as of US natives. Both immigrant groups had positive net contributions, meaning they paid more toward their private insurance coverage than they spent in receiving health services. Undocumented immigrants had an even higher net contribution—yes, undocumented immigrants get paychecks, and these paychecks have deductions. US natives had a negative net contribution, meaning that, per capita, their expenditures on health care were greater than their premiums.

These findings upend the common belief that immigrants are a drain on the US health care system. In reality, immigrants who contribute to Medicare and to private health insurers are subsidizing the health care of US citizens.

# REFERENCES

Crist C. US immigrants pay more for health insurance than they get in benefits. *Reuters*. October 10, 2018. https://www.reuters.com/article/us-health-insurance-immigrants/u-s-immigrants-pay-more-for-health-insurance-than-they-get-in-benefits-idUSKCN1MK24B Accessed September 13, 2019.

Figure from Zallman L, Woolhandler S, Touw S, Himmelstein D, Finnegan K. Immigrants pay more in private insurance premiums than they receive in benefits. *Health Affairs*. 2018; 37(10): 1663–68. doi: 10.1377/hlthaff.2018.0309. Reproduced with permission.

Zallman L, Woolhandler S, Himmelstein D, Bor D, McCormick D. Immigrants contributed an estimated $115.2 billion more to the Medicare Trust Fund than they took out in 2002–09. *Health Affairs*. 2013; 32(6):1153–60. doi: 10.1377/hlthaff.2012.1223

# [ 19 ]

# DYING YOUNG IN THE UNITED STATES

## CHILD MORTALITY IN THE UNITED STATES AND THE OECD19, BY AGE GROUP, 1960–2010

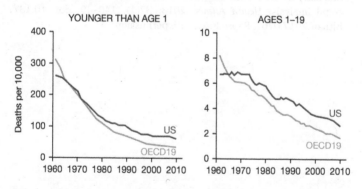

Child mortality is declining worldwide, according to a half-century's worth of data from the Human Mortality Database and the WHO. Since the 1980s, however, the United States has had higher rates of mortality for kids aged 0 to 19, compared to other wealthy Organization for Economic Cooperation and Development (OECD) nations. In 2013, UNICEF ranked the health and safety of children in the United States 25th out of 29 developed countries.

*Pained.* Michael D. Stein and Sandro Galea, Oxford University Press (2020). © Oxford University Press.
DOI: 10.1093/oso/9780197510384.001.0001

According to a 2018 *Health Affairs* study, from 2001 to 2010, the risk of death in the United States compared to peer nations was 76% greater for infants and 57% greater for children and youth age 1 to 19. In that same time frame, American teens age 15 to 19 were 82 times likelier to die from gun-related homicide.

US policymakers need to focus on preventing child mortality by preventing the largest contributors: perinatal deaths, car accidents, and firearm assaults. Healthy kids become healthy adults. We have a duty to create a world where every child is able to do so.

# REFERENCE

Figure from Thakrar AP, Forrest AD, Maltenfort MG, Forrest CB. Child mortality in the US and 19 OECD comparator nations: a 50-year time-trend analysis. *Health Affairs.* 2018; 37(1): 140–49. doi: 10.1377/hlthaff.2017.0767. Reproduced with permission.

# A SURE ARGUMENT

*Some health-related topics seem to provoke perennial disagreement. Vaccines and conspiracy theories, whether immigration is going to harm our health, whether we are doing enough for the health of our veterans, whether abortion should be part of providing health care— these arguments never seem to go away. But that does not mean we should not try to resolve them.*

# 20

# VACCINES AND CONSPIRACIES

Near the end of 2018, data released by the Centers for Disease Control and Prevention (CDC) showed that a small, but growing, number of children in the United States were not getting recommended vaccinations. One in 77 infants born in 2017 did not receive any vaccinations; that's more than four times as many unvaccinated children as the country had at the turn of the century. Some of this may be due to lack of access to vaccines; populations without insurance and those living in rural areas have greater rates of nonvaccination. But part of it is also likely due to the rise of conspiracy theories and the willful dismissal of scientific evidence when it comes to vaccines.

Vaccinations have always provoked anxiety. But the data on vaccines that are in widespread use are now clear: vaccines are safe and save lives. Nonetheless, conspiracism insists that we don't know all the facts, that things about vaccines are not as they seem. Conspiracism fuels the anti-vaccine movement, nudging people to accept anecdotes (e.g., "I heard about one child who got a measles vaccine and developed autism") over statistics.

And, with the unpredictability of political leaders' words and actions, we are one menacing sentence away from real public health trouble. Imagine if a president one day were to announce, "People

*Pained*. Michael D. Stein and Sandro Galea, Oxford University Press (2020). © Oxford University Press.
DOI: 10.1093/oso/9780197510384.001.0001

are saying that maybe we don't really need quite so many vaccines for our kids. After all, look at all this autism that's around." This vague conspiratorial phrasing—"people are saying"—this kind of innuendo, would immediately corrode confidence in our collective public health policy. Conspiracism undermines authority.

Conspiracists question the safety of vaccines not just because of distrust of the pharmaceutical industry, but because they tend to question the function of government itself. For them, vaccination policy raises questions about the scope and intentions of federal power. The growing avoidance of vaccination seems to reflect interlocking anxieties about media, science, and government. Yet no matter how passionately the conspiracists make their case, it remains true that universal vaccination is in our common interest. Unlike conspiracists, public health advocates adhere to standards of evidence and falsifiability; when conspiracists disregard explanation and refuse any form of correction, they place health at risk.

## REFERENCES

Mellerson JL, Maxwell CB, Knighton CL, Kriss JL, Seither R, Black CL. Vaccination Coverage for selected vaccines and exemption rates among children in kindergarten—United States, 2017–18 school year. *Morbidity and Mortality Weekly Report (MMWR)*. 2018; 67(40): 1115–22.

Sugerman DE, Barskey AE, Delea MG, et al. Measles outbreak in a highly vaccinated population, San Diego, 2008: role of the intentionally undervaccinated. *Pediatrics*. 2010; 125(4): 747–55. doi: 10.1542/peds.2009-1653

# 21

# HEALTH SYSTEMS AND PUBLIC HEALTH THINKING

Every health care provider—from pediatricians to geriatricians—has seen how homelessness affects health. The disordered lives of homeless patients disrupt appointment-keeping and medication adherence, even as they generate need for more treatment by driving health challenges like depression, high blood pressure, and hospitalizations.

Some health systems have begun to address the link between homelessness and health. One Boston health system, for example, announced plans to subsidize housing for the patients for whom it is accountable, to give this population some measure of the shelter and stability necessary for good health.

This is an example of a growing practice among health systems, which are beginning to address the foundational forces that shape health. Their reason for doing so is partly financial. For example, Medicaid, in some states, adjusts payments to hospitals based on whether a patient is homeless—homelessness is treated like any other complicating diagnosis, an additional cost of care. So health systems can lose money if they do not collect and appropriately bill for housing status. But there are also more charitable reasons for health systems' new focus, including the possibility that collecting information like homeless status can drive new program

*Pained*. Michael D. Stein and Sandro Galea, Oxford University Press (2020). © Oxford University Press.
DOI: 10.1093/oso/9780197510384.001.0001

development and position the health systems to help fix underlying economic and social problems, toward the ultimate goal of improving patients' health.

Perhaps, at core, health systems are addressing health at the level of root causes because they have to. As a society, we tend to forget that health is a public good supported by our collective investment in resources such as education, the environment, and, indeed, housing. Health systems can help us remember, by investing in these resources, to improve the health of patients.

In many ways, health systems taking on this new role is welcome. Health systems are ubiquitous, touching all our lives. Their administrators are in a position to take the lead on creating new approaches to health. But should the onus for doing so lie solely on them? Should health systems own and run food pantries, or manage apartment buildings? Should they take on the provision of social services as part of patient care? And, in pursuit of these new services, should they risk taking resources from diagnosis and treatment, hitherto the centerpieces of medical care? It seems self-evident that attempting to do all of this could place an undue burden on health systems and allow the responsibility of promoting health to drift from where it should really lie—on all of us. Health is our collective responsibility. Health systems can nudge us toward a better understanding of what truly shapes health, but it is ultimately our responsibility to act on that knowledge and build a world that generates health.

# 22

# MISCONCEPTIONS ABOUT
# VETERANS AND HEALTH

There are 200,000 new veterans each year, adding to the 20 million Americans who have served in the military. Nearly five decades since our military went all-volunteer, and after almost two decades of constant war, we continue to misunderstand the military. Novelists and moviemakers depict veterans who are disconnected and marginalized. That is largely not so. The military is solidly middle class, and in many ways it is a select group. High physical and educational standards—a high school degree required—means that 71% of young adults would fail to qualify if they tried to enlist. The military is also an ever more diverse group. Women now make up one in six enlisted, and both sexes are more ethnically diverse than the civilian population. Veterans are more likely to vote, volunteer, give to charity, and attend town meetings than nonveterans. Female and black veterans experience a wage premium (2% and 7%, respectively) over nonveterans.

The military, and veterans, therefore, increasingly represent a rapidly diversifying middle of the country. But the health of military and veterans highlights the challenges our soldiers face. Since the first Gulf War in 1990, veterans have had worse mortality than

*Pained.* Michael D. Stein and Sandro Galea, Oxford University Press (2020). © Oxford University Press.
DOI: 10.1093/oso/9780197510384.001.0001

the general population, due perhaps to multiple deployments and survival from injuries that would have killed soldiers in the past.

Aside from mortality, mental health problems are a particular concern. More soldiers kill themselves than are killed on our battlefields—20 a day, which is 50% higher than the civilian rate. The majority of these suicides are over 55 years old, although rates among younger veterans have been rising.

Beyond suicide, key mental health concerns among veterans include posttraumatic stress disorder (PTSD). Itself disruptive, PTSD foreshadows increased risks of physical health problems, substance use/misuse, homelessness, and violence. Less studied, but equally important, are high rates of depression and anxiety among veterans. Rates of chronic pain and physical disability rates are also unfortunately high. These challenges make the Veterans Health Administration's unique expertise in mental health care provision and rehabilitation services all the more crucial.

For these reasons, moves to privatize veterans' health care and narrow access to these services do veterans a disservice, shortchanging a fundamental social contract. Soldiers protect us and keep us safe; we owe it to them to provide the best possible care when they finish their service. Their health is the public's health.

## REFERENCES

CNN Library. Department of Veterans Affairs Fast Facts. *CNN*. September 20, 2018. https://www.cnn.com/2014/05/30/us/department-of-veterans-affairs-fast-facts/index.html Accessed September 13, 2019.

Fox M, Horch A. 3 ways military veterans can successfully transition into the civilian workforce. *CNBC*. July 26, 2019. https://www.cnbc.com/2019/07/25/how-veterans-can-successfully-transition-into-the-civilian-workforce.html Accessed September 13, 2019.

Shane III L. VA: Suicide rate for younger veterans increased by more than 10%. *Military Times*. September 26, 2018. https://www.militarytimes.

com/news/pentagon-congress/2018/09/26/suicide-rate-spikes-among-younger-veterans/ Accessed September 13, 2019.

Wentling N. VA reveals its veteran suicide statistic included active-duty troops. *Stars and Stripes*. June 20, 2018. https://www.stripes.com/news/us/va-reveals-its-veteran-suicide-statistic-included-active-duty-troops-1.533992 Accessed September 13, 2019.

# [ 23 ]

# IMMIGRATION AND
# THE HEALTH OF THE PUBLIC

Immigration is neither a new issue nor an exclusively American one. In 2017, there were more than 250 million immigrants living worldwide, and about 2.4 million people migrate across national borders each year. Migration also occurs within national borders—it is estimated that more than 750 million people live within their country of birth, but in a different region. Economic, political, and social forces drive migration. Migrants who are forced to leave their country due to war or persecution become refugees; there were over 65 million refugees worldwide at the end of 2017.

The health of immigrants in their adopted home is strongly shaped by social, economic, and political conditions in that country. Legal status in the host country, for example, is associated with access to a broad range of health services and resultant better health. A study in Denmark found that while refugees were disadvantaged in terms of some cardiovascular disease outcomes, and equal or better off than a Danish-born comparison group in others, family-reunified immigrants had significantly lower incidence of stroke, cardiovascular disease, and myocardial infarction across the board.

*Pained*. Michael D. Stein and Sandro Galea, Oxford University Press (2020). © Oxford University Press.
DOI: 10.1093/oso/9780197510384.001.0001

Perhaps unsurprisingly, aggressive anti-immigration policies create poor health for the population they target. For example, family separation and detention at our borders traumatize families, deepening the mental health needs of this vulnerable group. And federal raids can affect the birthweight of babies born to US-born Latina women, following immigration authority raids in search of undocumented Latinos.

Creating the conditions for immigrants to stay healthy helps us all. Consider: a measles outbreak in Minnesota was fueled by low vaccination rates among refugees, who often mistrust health providers and fear discrimination and deportation. Ultimately, this outbreak—caused by the conditions of marginalization faced by immigrants—threatened the health of everyone, immigrant and native-born alike. Policies which further marginalize immigrant communities can increase this risk. Rather than listen to voices that rail against the imagined evils of immigration, we should do all we can as a country to maximize the health of immigrants, by working to include them in the fabric of American life and providing them with the basic social services they need in order to be well.

# REFERENCES

31 people are newly displaced every minute of the day. United Nations High Commissioner for Refugees Web site. https://www.unhcr.org/global-trends2017/. Accessed September 13, 2019.

Byberg S, Agyemang C, Zwisler A, Krasnik A, Norredam M. Cardiovascular disease incidence and survival: Are migrants always worse off? *European Journal of Epidemiology*. 2016; 31(7): 667–77. doi: 10.1007/s10654-015-0024-7

Department of Economic and Social Affairs: Population. United Nations Web site. https://www.un.org/en/development/desa/population/publications/technical/index.asp. Accessed September 13, 2019.

International Migration 2017. United Nations Web site. https://www.un.org/en/development/desa/population/migration/publications/wallchart/docs/MigrationWallChart2017.pdf. Accessed September 13, 2019.

Mole B. Anti-vaccine advocates appointed to Minnesota autism council after measles outbreak. *Ars Technica*. January 25, 2019. https://arstechnica.com/science/2019/01/anti-vaccine-advocates-appointed-to-minnesota-autism-council-after-measles-outbreak/. Accessed September 13, 2019.

Novak NL, Geronimus AT, Martinez-Cardoso AM. Change in birth outcomes among infants born to Latina mothers after a major immigration raid. *International Journal of Epidemiology*. 2017; 46(3): 839–49. doi: 10.1093/ije/dyw346

Shah A. Immigration. Global Issues Web site. http://www.globalissues.org/article/537/immigration Accessed September 13, 2019.

Sousa E, Agudelo-Suárez A, Benavides FG, et al. Immigration, work and health in Spain: The influence of legal status and employment contract on reported health indicators. *International Journal of Public Health*. 2010; 55(5): 443–51. doi: 10.1007/s00038-010-0141-8

# [ 24 ]

# OUT OF SCHOOL, OUT OF LUCK

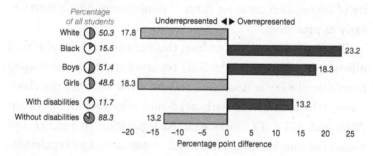

Students Suspended from School Compared to Student Population, by Race, Sex, and Disability Status, School Year 2013–14

Out-of-school suspension is linked to lower grades, increased expulsions, and increased risk of incarceration. Disciplinary actions are often distributed unequally, based on gender, race, and personal ability. At the request of Congress, the US Government Accountability Office (GAO) reviewed disciplinary patterns across schools. As shown in the figure, although black students account for only 15.5% of the K–12 student population, they make up 39% of the nation's suspensions. Boys are also overrepresented in out-of-school suspensions, as are students living with a disability.

*Pained*. Michael D. Stein and Sandro Galea, Oxford University Press (2020). © Oxford University Press.
DOI: 10.1093/oso/9780197510384.001.0001

Disciplinary action through suspension is centered on a student's behavior, which is often influenced by complex social challenges such as poverty, mental illness, and lack of parental support. Most suspensions result from multiple school absences and tardy reports, which are commonly linked to difficult family situations. Chronic tardiness most affects low-income students, who often care for younger siblings or work to support their family. Furthermore, teachers' implicit biases also contribute to the harshness of the punishment they dispense. Research shows that students of color suffer from harsher disciplinary outcomes from white teachers than from teachers of the same race. And boys and black students make up the majority of suspension cases—a form of punishment which starts as early as preschool.

There are ways we can address this unfairness. Several school officials interviewed by the GAO reported trying to move away from disciplinary actions that remove children from the classroom, which interfere with academic achievement. Between 2016 and 2017, 17 states enacted legislation to restrict and reduce the number of out-of-school suspensions and expulsions. An elementary school official in Georgia reported that they no longer discipline based on tardiness. Schools in Massachusetts have attempted to collaborate with mental health professionals and social workers, to support students undergoing traumatic experiences. Districts in Texas have introduced "personal break rooms" where children can calm down and redirect their emotions after a frustrating incident. These are examples of how we can address students' behavior, while reducing the inequalities that can influence disciplinary actions. Such steps can help create better learning environments, with the aim of producing healthier students.

# REFERENCES

Child well-being: key considerations for policymakers, including the need for a federal cross-agency priority goal. Government Accountability Office Web site. https://www.gao.gov/assets/690/688252.pdf Accessed September 13, 2019.

Cuellar AE, Markowitz S. School suspension and the school-to-prison pipeline. *International Review of Law and Economics*. 2015; 43: 98–106.

Discipline disparities. National Clearinghouse on Supportive School Discipline Web site. https://supportiveschooldiscipline.org/learn/reference-guides/discipline-disparities Accessed September 13, 2019.

Fabelo T, Thompson M, Plotkin M, Carmichael D, Marchbanks III M, Booth E. *Breaking schools' rules: a statewide study of how school discipline relates to students' success and juvenile justice involvement*; 2011. https://csgjusticecenter.org/wp-content/uploads/2012/08/Breaking_Schools_Rules_Report_Final.pdf Accessed September 13, 2019.

Figure from K–12 education: discipline disparities for black students, boys, and students with disabilities. Government Accountability Office Web site. https://www.gao.gov/assets/700/690828.pdf Accessed September 13, 2019.

Lindsay CA, Hart CMD. Teacher race and school discipline. *Education Next*. 2017; 17(1): 72–78.

Policy snapshot: suspension and expulsion. Education Commission of the States Web site. https://www.ecs.org/wp-content/uploads/Suspension_and_Expulsion.pdf Accessed September 13, 2019.

# PSEUDOSCIENCE AND ABORTION POLICY

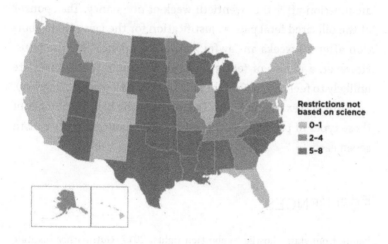

Restrictions not
based on science
■ 0–1
■ 2–4
■ 5–8

In 2012, when US Representative Todd Akin from Missouri
was asked if abortion was justified in cases of rape, he notoriously said that pregnancy as a result of rape is rare because "the
female body has ways to try and shut that whole thing down."
Arguments made against abortion, like this one, are often riddled
with pseudoscience.

As the attached map shows, 29 states, home to 88 million
women, have implemented at least two, state-wide abortion
restrictions not backed by scientific evidence.

*Pained.* Michael D. Stein and Sandro Galea, Oxford University Press (2020). © Oxford University Press.
DOI: 10.1093/oso/9780197510384.001.0001

For example, Texas's "A Woman's Right to Know" booklet, offered to patients before having an abortion, uses deceptive language to lead readers to believe that abortion increases the risk of breast cancer. *The Washington Post*'s Fact Checker gave this claim in the booklet three "Pinocchios" on their rating scale, meaning that there was a "significant factual error" present. The American College of Obstetricians and Gynecologists released a statement in 2009 concluding that there is "no association between induced abortion and breast cancer."

Kentucky's Senate Bill 5, passed in 2017, made it illegal to have an abortion after the twentieth week of pregnancy. The sponsor of the bill cited fetal pain as justification for the law, calling abortion after 20 weeks an "awful painful experience" for the fetus. However, a review of fetal pain evidence found that fetuses are unlikely to feel pain before the third trimester (around 29 weeks).

Kansas, Texas, and South Dakota have the highest number of these types of pseudoscientific information policies in place, with seven each.

# REFERENCES

Figure from states hostile to abortion rights, 2017. Guttmacher Institute Web site. https://www.guttmacher.org/infographic/2018/states-hostile-abortion-rights-2017 Accessed September 14, 2019

Induced abortion and breast cancer risk. American College of Obstetricians and Gynecologists Web site. https://www.acog.org/Clinical-Guidance-and-Publications/Committee-Opinions/Committee-on-Gynecologic-Practice/Induced-Abortion-and-Breast-Cancer-Risk Accessed September 14, 2019.

Jaco C. Jaco report: full interview with Todd Akin. KTVI FOX 2 News St. Louis Web site. https://fox2now.com/2012/08/19/the-jaco-report-august-19-2012/ Published August 19, 2012. Accessed September 14, 2019.

Kentucky General Assembly Web site. https://legislature.ky.gov/Pages/index.aspx Accessed September 14, 2019.

Kessler G. About the Fact Checker. *The Washington Post*. January 1, 2017. https://beta.washingtonpost.com/politics/2019/01/07/about-fact-checker/ Accessed September 14, 2019.

Lee M. Texas state booklet misleads women on abortions and their risk of breast cancer. *The Washington Post*. December 14, 2016. https://www.washingtonpost.com/news/fact-checker/wp/2016/12/14/texas-state-booklet-misleads-women-on-abortions-and-their-risk-of-breast-cancer/ Accessed September 14, 2019.

Lee SJ, Ralston HJ, Drey EA, Partridge JC, Rosen MA. Fetal pain: a systematic multidisciplinary review of the evidence. *JAMA: The Journal of the American Medical Association*. 2005; 294(8): 947–54. doi: 10.1001/jama.294.8.947

Nash E, Gold R, Mohammed L, Ansari-Thomas Z, Cappello O. Policy trends in the states, 2017. Guttmacher Institute Web site. https://www.guttmacher.org/article/2018/01/policy-trends-states-2017 Published January 2, 2018. Accessed September 14, 2019.

Smith J. Kentucky's new fetal pain law, like most abortion restrictions, is based on junk science. *The Intercept*. January 22, 2017. https://theintercept.com/2017/01/22/kentuckys-new-fetal-pain-law-like-most-abortion-restrictions-is-based-on-junk-science/ Accessed September 14, 2019.

A Woman's right to know. Texas Department of State Health Services Web site. https://dshs.texas.gov/wrtk/ Accessed September 14, 2019.

# SECTION 5

# FOLLOW THE MONEY

*We spend more money on health than all other high-income countries, yet our health indicators remain terrible. Ultimately, we are spending on the wrong things; unless we pay attention to the health of the poorest 50% of Americans, and then invest in improving the conditions that shape the health of all, we will continue to get sick.*

# [ 26 ]

# INCOME INEQUALITY AND
# OUR HEALTH

Pretax incomes for the poorest 50% of Americans have stayed mostly unchanged for the past 40 years, widening income gaps in the country. We leave the question of why inequality matters for the economy to others. What is of concern to us is whether income inequality matters to our health, and, to the extent that it does, how the health profession should respond.

In 1992, Richard Wilkinson, then a professor at the University of Sussex, published a paper in *The British Medical Journal* called "Income distribution and life expectancy." The paper concerned 12 European countries and concluded that "the relation between income distribution and life expectancy is sufficiently strong to produce significant associations." The paper's provocative thesis launched two decades of intense scientific discussion about the influence of national income inequality on health (and death), including several systematic reviews and books. This work, which continues to the present day, shows that income inequality is a foundational driver of physical and mental health. By way of example, a 2018 systematic review considers the relationship between income inequality and depression, and it concludes that across studies there is "greater risk of depression in populations

*Pained*. Michael D. Stein and Sandro Galea, Oxford University Press (2020). © Oxford University Press.
DOI: 10.1093/oso/9780197510384.001.0001

with higher income inequality relative to populations with lower inequality."

Why might income inequality affect the health of the public?

Countries or regions where there are wide gaps in income tend to be characterized by weaker social ties and less investment in the social and physical resources that create health. Countries with more income inequality are less likely to have healthy air, water, and food, safe places to work and play, and affordable quality housing—all of which are necessary for health.

For these reasons, income inequality should be a core focus of public health. It is true that discussing subjects like taxation policies, the minimum wage, and universal income guarantees broadens the scope of what we are used to discussing in the context of health. However, broadening the conversation in this way has long been a first step toward creating a healthier world. After all, at one time, few imagined that cigarettes had anything to do with health, and even doctors promoted smoking. It took a widening of our collective imagination to see tackling smoking and the tobacco industry as central to promoting health. In the same way, by discussing income inequality, we start to see the truth of what the data are telling us: money—who has it and who does not—is at the heart of health in our society. Until we address this, we will continue to see health gaps between those at the top of the economic ladder and those at the bottom.

## REFERENCES

Ashkenas J. Nine new findings about inequality in the United States. *The New York Times*. December 16, 2016. https://www.nytimes.com/interactive/2016/12/16/business/economy/nine-new-findings-about-income-inequality-piketty.html?auth=login-email Accessed September 16, 2019.

Krugman P. Why inequality matters. *The New York Times*. December 15, 2013. https://www.nytimes.com/2013/12/16/opinion/krugman-why-inequality-matters.html?mtrref=www.google.com&assetType=opinion Accessed September 16, 2019.

Lawrence L. Cigarettes were once "physician" tested, approved. Healio Web site. https://www.healio.com/hematology-oncology/news/print/hemonc-today/%7B241d62a7-fe6e-4c5b-9fed-a33cc6e4bd7c%7D/cigarettes-were-once-physician-tested-approved Published March 10, 2019. Accessed September 16, 2019.

Lynch J, Smith GD, Harper S, et al. Is Income Inequality a Determinant of Population Health? Part 1. A Systematic Review. *The Milbank Quarterly*. 2004; 82(1): 5–99.

Patel V, Burns JK, Dhingra M, Tarver L, Kohrt BA, Lund C. Income inequality and depression: a systematic review and meta-analysis of the association and a scoping review of mechanisms. *World Psychiatry*. 2018; 17(1): 76–89. doi: 10.1002/wps.20492

Wilkinson RG. Income distribution and life expectancy. *The BMJ*. 1992; 304(6820): 165–68.

Wilkinson R, Pickett K. *The spirit level: why greater equality makes societies stronger*. New York, NY: Bloomsbury Press; 2009.

# CAN CEOS SAVE THE HEALTH OF AMERICANS?

The health of Americans is not what it should be. In the United States, we die younger and live unhealthier lives than populations of high-income peer countries. Into this breach of poor health have rushed many efforts to address this challenge. These efforts are informed by a range of motivations, from a genuine interest in creating healthier populations, to a desire to seize a commercial opportunity, to a combination of these aims. These moves include health system consolidation and the efforts of large corporations such as Amazon and Walmart to reinvent care delivery. Underlying private sector efforts to transform health care is an assumption that CEOs, accountable to shareholders rather than to communities, may transform health care more quickly and thoroughly than the public sector has, or perhaps can. But is there reason to believe that CEOs, and the private sector, are able to this?

Over the past 50 years, the cultural reputation of the corporate CEO has soared. The "right" CEO, we are told, can dramatically improve a private company's performance. We have since extrapolated this belief to include executives operating in

*Pained*. Michael D. Stein and Sandro Galea, Oxford University Press (2020). © Oxford University Press.
DOI: 10.1093/oso/9780197510384.001.0001

the public sector—a gifted principal can transform a school, for example, or a top manager can take an NGO to new heights. But the evidence that the CEO and the private sector can actually be a force for good health remains dubious.

In the 1980s, as the British government decentralized its health care management model, CEOs were given full responsibility for the administration and performance of individual public hospitals. Under this system, individual hospital boards could now select and reward individual CEOs. Frequent movements of CEOs seeking salary increases across British hospitals followed, providing an ideal setting to study whether CEOs improved hospital performance. A study found that, while a CEO could affect certain aspects of her or his environment—growth in the number of beds, for example, or job satisfaction of staff—the person at the top did not affect health outcomes.

In some ways this shouldn't have come as a surprise. Hospitals are wildly complex. They entail thousands of diagnoses, thousands of procedures or "products." A CEO, even if she is a physician, cannot keep up with all her products, and so, in a sense, is flying blind. Here in the United States—where the success of "star" health system CEOs has never been proven—there is the added difficulty that payment for service is dependent on external forces, in particular contracts with insurers.

This points to the real problem with a CEO takeover of health care: achieving better health depends on much more than the conditions that drive the fiscal well-being of a single organization, that is, the conditions over which the CEO has the most influence. The truly important conditions are social, economic, and environmental. Improving these conditions as a means of improving health takes time and effort across a range of sectors, both public and private. A good CEO can be a welcome and important part of these efforts, but best functions as a supporting player, rather than as the focal point of what is, at heart, a collective effort.

## REFERENCE

1. Janke K, Propper C, Sadun R. The impact of CEOs in the public sector: evidence from the NHS. NBER Working Paper 25853. May 2019.

# [ 28 ]

# THE HEALTH OF THE POOREST 50%

No relationship is more clearly established in population health science than the one between income and health. Those among us who are fortunate enough to have higher income live longer, healthier lives. By way of example, those born in 1960 who are in the lowest income quintile, can expect to live till age 76; those in the highest income quintile can expect to live till age 89. Money buys access to the resources that create a healthier life, from safe neighborhoods to walk in, to clean air to breathe, to time off to care for our children when they are sick, to nutritious food. We write about this today, not because it is news, but because, quite simply, the United States is on the brink of creating a class of permanent health have-nots, shaped by entrenched class divides and ever-increasing income disparity.

As partially noted in chapter 26, pretax income for the poorest 50% of Americans has remained the same over the past 40 years, while their after-tax income has dropped as taxes have increased for this same group. Regressive taxation has deepened wealth gaps, virtually assuring a continuing cycle of low income earning. The national share of income owned by the richest 50% of Americans has grown commensurately during this period, and our health indicators have responded accordingly. The slope of the

*Pained*. Michael D. Stein and Sandro Galea, Oxford University Press (2020). © Oxford University Press.
DOI: 10.1093/oso/9780197510384.001.0001 .

income–health relationship has grown even steeper since 2000; the health advantage that those with higher incomes have over those with lower incomes is greater than it has been in the past four or more decades. Going back to the example we started with, for those born in 1930, the poorest quintile could expect to live till age 77, the richest quintile until 82. The life expectancy gap has widened from 5 to 13 years. The rich have gained years while the poor have not.

Why is this? We as a country continue to invest less in the social resources that can mitigate the challenges that come with a lower income, even as we spend ever more on high-end medicine that is accessed principally by those who can afford it. Social institutions like education that traditionally have led to social mobility and better health have become increasingly the provenance of the well-off.

That about one out of every two Americans now has health and survival outcomes no better—and potentially worse—than those born decades earlier is alarming. Should this not be on the front page of every newspaper every day?

## REFERENCES

Ashkenas J. Nine new findings about inequality in the United States. *The New York Times*. December 16, 2016. https://www.nytimes.com/interactive/2016/12/16/business/economy/nine-new-findings-about-income-inequality-piketty.html?auth=login-email Accessed September 16, 2019.

Bor J, Cohen GH, Galea S. Population health in an era of rising income inequality: USA, 1980—2015. *The Lancet*. 2017; 389(10077): 1475–1490.

Fletcher H. Dr. Tony Iton: "What's in the way of the American dream right now?" *BirdDog*. March 21, 2018. https://readbirddog.com/2018/03/21/dr-tony-iton-on-why-american-dream-is-faltering/ Accessed September 16, 2019.

Indicators of higher education equity in the United States. The Pell Institute for the Study of Opportunity in Higher Education Web site. http://pellinstitute.org/indicators/ Accessed September 16, 2019.

Opportunity Insights Web site. https://opportunityinsights.org Accessed September 16, 2019.

# 29

# CAN WE PROMOTE PUBLIC HEALTH AND GENERATE RETURN ON OUR INVESTMENT?

It is widely recognized that the United States spends far more on health—or, more accurately, on medical care—than any other country on earth. This leads to a considerable amount of hand-wringing, and also some well-considered ideas about how we can spend our money better. While most thinking about how we may best rethink our health spending features some acknowledgment that we should spend more on prevention, our health investment remains resolutely focused on curative care. Of the $3.3 trillion we spent on health in 2016, only about 2% was spent on classic public health activities, such as disease monitoring and surveillance.

Does this spending truly reflect what we want for our lives and health? Was Benjamin Franklin not correct, when he wrote, "An ounce of prevention is worth a pound of cure"? To put it more prosaically—as great as it would be to live in a world where we could cure a terrible disease like Alzheimer's, would it not be better to live in a world where such a disease did not exist?

*Pained*. Michael D. Stein and Sandro Galea, Oxford University Press (2020). © Oxford University Press.
DOI: 10.1093/oso/9780197510384.001.0001

Perhaps we spend more on cure than we do on prevention because we believe keeping people healthy is too expensive. But is this true? An analysis set out to assess the return on investment for high-income countries that adopt efforts to improve health. The authors conducted a systematic review of nearly 3,000 papers. They found that the median return on investment for public health interventions was 14 to 1—that is, for every dollar invested, it yields the same dollar back and another 14. They found that the more these interventions were established at the wider, national level, the higher the return, rising up to about 40 to 1 for the best investments.

What are these interventions? They include vaccination programs, taxes on sugar-sweetened beverages, building better cities to reduce falls, and early youth interventions to limit teenage pregnancy and delinquency. In other words, classic efforts to promote the public's health by shaping the conditions in which we live. If we could improve the public's health and improve our bottom line by investing in such efforts, then why do we not do so with greater regularity and commitment? We should not let inertia prolong the long-standing mismatch in this country between what we invest in and what actually makes us healthy.

## REFERENCES

Emanuel EJ. How can the United States spend its health care dollars better? *JAMA: The Journal of the American Medical Association*. 2016; 316(24): 2604–6. doi: 10.1001/jama.2016.16739

Galea S. An unhealthy mismatch. *The Milbank Quarterly*. 2017; 95(3): 486–9. doi: 10.1111/1468-0009.12275

Masters R, Anwar E, Collins B, Cookson R, Capewell S. Return on investment of public health interventions: a systematic review. *Journal of Epidemiology and Community Health*. 2017; 71(8): 827–34. doi: 10.1136/jech-2016-208141

The nation's health dollar ($3.5 trillion), calendar year 2017; where it came from. Centers for Medicare & Medicaid Services Web site. https://www.cms.gov/Research-Statistics-Data-and-Systems/Statistics-Trends-and-Reports/NationalHealthExpendData/Downloads/PieChartSourcesExpenditures.pdf Accessed September 17, 2019.

Squires D. US health care from a global perspective. The Commonwealth Fund Web site. https://www.commonwealthfund.org/publications/issue-briefs/2015/oct/us-health-care-global-perspective?redirect_source=/publications/issue-briefs/2015/oct/us-health-care-from-a-global-perspective Published October 8, 2015. Accessed September 17, 2019.

# 30

# THE POOR
# PEOPLE'S CAMPAIGN

Over 50 years ago, Martin Luther King Jr.'s ambitious project, the Poor People's Campaign, ended. In 1968, Dr. King had encouraged the civil rights movement to broaden its mission and demand full employment, housing, guaranteed basic income, and "an economic bill of rights." The plight of the impoverished, Dr. King knew, crosses racial lines, and the Poor People's Campaign was purposefully multiracial. Dr. King also knew poverty, like civil rights, is a moral issue and should be addressed with the same urgency as other forms of societal injustice.

Few would argue that poverty is indeed a moral issue. Yet taking the political steps to address poverty as a moral crisis remains controversial, polarizing Americans. This is likely, in part, because we have trouble conceptualizing the effects of poverty. We understand it is harmful, but we struggle to talk about it in a way that expresses the full scope of its harm and points toward workable solutions.

The key to discussing poverty lies in addressing its effect on health. Public health data accumulated since Dr. King's death might allow us to change the conversation about poverty and to show, in clear terms, how this crisis affects our health. If we can agree that poverty is a public health problem, we can address it

*Pained*. Michael D. Stein and Sandro Galea, Oxford University Press (2020). © Oxford University Press.
DOI: 10.1093/oso/9780197510384.001.0001

with public health solutions—that is to say, with the large-scale political commitment we have historically been able to muster to solve other problems that threaten our health.

Seen through the lens of health, the consequences of poverty are stark. The gap in life expectancy between the richest 20% and the poorest 20% of American men is nearly 15 years. Hundreds of thousands of deaths each year are linked to poverty-related causes. Those with low incomes have higher rates of accidents, injuries, depression, diabetes, substance use—the list goes on. The data are clear: poverty kills. When we accept this, we can then take the steps necessary to safeguard our health. We know that life expectancy for those with the lowest incomes can be improved by government expenditures. We must invest in the communities that need it most, using creative, compassion-informed policymaking to uplift the millions of Americans currently suffering. We should do this not just for the moral reasons Dr. King enumerated, but for the simple fact that the health of some is linked to the health of all. As long as we tolerate poverty, and the poor health it creates, our own health will remain tenuous.

If we do nothing, the problem of poverty will not only persist; it will likely worsen. Currently, the gap between health haves and health have-nots, directly mapping onto those who are wealthy and those who are poor, has widened in this country. Facing this emergency, we must insist on a conversation around poverty and health. No political candidate or party should be allowed to ignore the subject. While the moral argument against poverty remains robust, a public health perspective lends heft to our efforts to tackle poverty, and it should be front and center in all national discussions of this issue.

# REFERENCE

1. Chetty R, Stepner M, Abraham S, et al. The association between income and life expectancy in the United States, 2001—2014. *JAMA: The Journal of the American Medical Association*. 2016; 315(16): 1750–66. doi: 10.1001/jama.2016.4226

# 31

# SPENDING TOO MUCH ON THE WRONG THINGS

Americans spend half as many days in hospital as persons living in other high-income countries. We take fewer pills per person. We have fewer doctors per capita. Yet we spend two to three times as much on health care as other countries, and we have poorer health outcomes. In 2017, for example, we spent $3.5 trillion. Why? Because we overpay.

If spending equals utilization times price, then we can reduce the amount we spend by reducing either utilization or price. In a care delivery system that is already quite lean, utilization is hard to ratchet down much further. Certainly, we can better coordinate care when an ill person transitions between facilities. And we can cut back on unnecessary or repetitive testing. But if there is ever to be any real prospect of reducing our national spending, the main action has to be on price. Yet when any policymaker mentions price control, everyone looks away, and the conversation swings back to utilization, about reducing the number of "super-utilizers," or else we discuss "value," the newest buzzword.

Talking about overspending suggests that certain partners in the health system are charging more than they should. Since

*Pained*. Michael D. Stein and Sandro Galea, Oxford University Press (2020). © Oxford University Press.
DOI: 10.1093/oso/9780197510384.001.0001

about one third of our health care spending is related to hospitals (equipment, supplies) and another 20% is paid to health care providers, these are the obvious culprits. A 2003 *Health Affairs* study noted that the difference between health care spending in the United States and other countries "is caused mostly by higher prices for health care goods and services in the United States." This was reinforced in a 2018 paper that concluded much the same thing.

Health care spending is expected to rise more than 5% annually through the next decade, or about 1 percentage point faster than economic growth. Because we overpay for goods and services, it will become increasingly difficult to pay for programs like Medicare and Medicaid, and for employers to keep financing medical coverage for workers and their families.

But there will be a massive fallout if we spend less. Workers (employed by hospitals and medical device companies and pharmaceutical firms and doctor groups) will lose jobs if prices (hence payments) go down, and these medical jobs now drive the economies of large cities and small rural towns alike.

But are we getting our money's worth under the current system? Our health outcomes are inferior to those of Canada and European nations. If we spent less on hospitals and clinicians, we could spend more on the social services required to prevent or reduce illness, to make our entire population healthier. Would that not be worth the price of taking a long, hard look at our spending?

# REFERENCES

Anderson GF, Reinhardt UE, Hussey PS, Petrosyan V. It's the prices, stupid: Why the United States is so different from other countries. *Health Affairs.* 2003; 22(3): 89–105.

Papanicolas I, Woskie LR, Jha AK. Health care spending in the United States and other high-income countries. *JAMA: The Journal of the American Medical Association.* 2018; 319(10): 1024–39. doi: 10.1001/jama.2018.1150

# 32

# CLARIFYING
# MEDICAL BANKRUPTCY

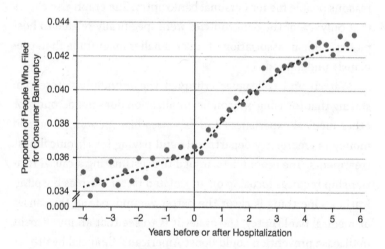

Medical bankruptcy is a much-debated topic, with most questions focused on exactly how many people file for it and how often it occurs. In 2005, Elizabeth Warren and her colleagues found medical costs led to over 40% of bankruptcies in the United States. This was followed by an update in 2009, pushing the proportion of bankruptcies due to medical expenses to 62%.

The Consumer Financial Protection Bureau's 2014 report conflicts with this causal attribution, citing that less than 1% of adults

*Pained.* Michael D. Stein and Sandro Galea, Oxford University Press (2020). © Oxford University Press.
DOI: 10.1093/oso/9780197510384.001.0001

in the United States file for bankruptcy, even though 20% of the population has great medical debt. In 2018, a group of economists reexamined this issue, concerned that the discrepancies in statistics were causing a misunderstanding of the problem. They studied a group of patients at a California hospital and looked at how hospital visits related to bankruptcy timing.

The figure shows an increase in people filing for bankruptcy after hospitalization, particularly between 1 and 4 years after admission. The researchers suggest that paying for medical bills out of pocket, and losing income because of missed work, are key reasons people file for personal bankruptcy. The graph also shows that only 4% of the bankruptcies were specifically related to hospitalization, an association of much smaller magnitude than previously understood.

Warren and colleagues critiqued the economists' research, stating that focusing only on hospitalization does not account for other medical experiences and expenses like spending time and money in emergency departments and paying for chronic illness treatments. The economists argued that estimating a causal relationship requires focusing on an isolated factor, such as hospitalization. One thing is clear: the better we understand the causes of medical bankruptcy, the easier it is to see that an investment in disease prevention could boost Americans' financial health, as well as their physical and mental well-being.

## REFERENCES

Figure from Dobkin C, Finkelstein A, Kluender R, Notowidigdo MJ. Myth and measurement: the case of medical bankruptcies. *The New England Journal of Medicine*. 2018; 378(12): 1076–8. Reproduced with permission.

Himmelstein DU, Woolhandler S, Warren E. Myth and measurement: the case of medical bankruptcies. *The New England Journal of Medicine*. 2018; 378(23): 2245–6. doi: 10.1056/NEJMc1805444

Sanger-Katz M. Elizabeth Warren and a scholarly debate over medical bankruptcy that won't go away. *The New York Times*. June 6, 2018. https://www.nytimes.com/2018/06/06/upshot/elizabeth-warren-and-a-scholarly-debate-over-medical-bankruptcy-that-wont-go-away.html Accessed September 17, 2019.

# 33

# HIGH PAY GETS HIGHER, LOW PAY GETS LOWER

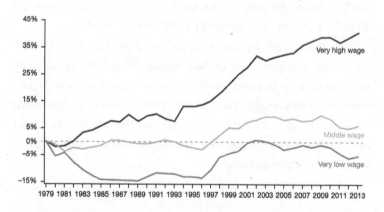

An employed person in the United States is healthier than an unemployed person, and a highly paid employee is likelier to have better health. As of this writing, the federal minimum wage in the United States is set at $7.25 per hour. Workers who receive tips are required to receive a minimum of $2.13 per hour. These minimums have not been changed since 2009 and 1996, respectively.

A 2018 health policy brief in *Health Affairs* highlights fluctuations in wages and how population health reflects these changes. In the brief, J. Paul Leigh and Juan Du emphasize that the labor market does not strictly follow basic economic assumptions. In

*Pained.* Michael D. Stein and Sandro Galea, Oxford University Press (2020). © Oxford University Press.
DOI: 10.1093/oso/9780197510384.001.0001

particular, an increase in wages may not reduce quantity or quality of work, as an economist critiquing minimum wage hikes might expect. Instead, the study's authors argue increased wages can improve productivity by boosting morale.

Wages between 1979 and 2013 rose notably only for those with very high pay. As the figure depicts, people in the middle wage group have not seen much of an increase in pay over the years, barely reaching a 10% increase in 2009.

Those with very low wages have almost exclusively seen drops in their pay over the decades. In the United States, low-wage workers make up 29% of the workforce. This means there are 47 million people who are paid poorly for their work.

The study authors also explain how increases in the minimum wage can positively impact health, citing prior research on the connections to lower smoking, fewer missed work days, and improved birthweight. With many states looking to raise their minimum wages, the authors recommend that those still caught in the debate should approach the decision from both a health and economic perspective.

# REFERENCES

Doyle A. 2019 federal and state minimum wage rates. The Balance Careers Web site. https://www.thebalancecareers.com/2018-19-federal-state-minimum-wage-rates-2061043 Accessed September 17, 2019.

Employment strongly influences health. The Pew Charitable Trusts Web site. https://www.pewtrusts.org/en/research-and-analysis/data-visualizations/2018/employment-strongly-influences-health Accessed September 17, 2019.

Figure from Leigh JP, Du J. Effects of minimum wages on population health. *Health Affairs* Health Policy Brief. https://www.healthaffairs.org/do/10.1377/hpb20180622.107025/full/ Published October 4, 2018. Accessed September 17, 2019. Reproduced with permission.

Lenhart O. The impact of minimum wages on population health: evidence from 24 OECD countries. *The European Journal of Health Economics.* 2017; 18(8): 1031–9. doi: 10.1007/s10198-016-0847-5

Minimum wage tracker. Economic Policy Institute Web site. https://www.epi.org/minimum-wage-tracker/ Accessed September 17, 2019.

Witters D. Employed Americans in better health than the unemployed. Gallup Web site. https://news.gallup.com/poll/155408/employed-americans-better-health-unemployed.aspx Published June 29, 2012. Accessed September 17, 2019.

# DARK THOUGHTS

*In 2018, the National Center for Health Statistics reported that, between 2016 and 2017, US life expectancy dropped from 78.7 to 78.6 years. That marked the third consecutive year that life expectancy in the United States has decreased. This makes for dark thoughts. How does one talk about pain, opioids, violence, guns, mental illness— markers of despair—in a way that points toward solutions to these problems?*

# 34

# THE STORY WE ARE NOT TALKING ABOUT ENOUGH

In 1918, a pandemic of Spanish flu infected approximately one third of the global population, killing between 20 and 50 million people. In the United States alone, more than 650,000 people died, enough to contribute to a decline in the country's life expectancy. For a century, this was the worst decline in American health, until, in 2018, the National Center for Health Statistics reported that, between 2016 and 2017, US life expectancy dropped from 78.7 to 78.6 years—the third consecutive year life expectancy in the United States has declined. Yet, somehow, these data were not headline news every day for weeks after their release. They did not move instantly to the center of our national discourse. The stir they caused was decidedly minor.

What accounts for our lack of attention to this news? Perhaps we have simply accepted our poor health. Maybe we have decided we can live with a trend in which US life expectancy lags relative to other economically comparable countries.

Perhaps, then, we believe our collective poor health is not our individual problem. Sure, we think, our neighbors may face addiction, suicide, and depression, but we can avoid this fate in our

*Pained*. Michael D. Stein and Sandro Galea, Oxford University Press (2020). © Oxford University Press.
DOI: 10.1093/oso/9780197510384.001.0001

own lives by making the right choices about health and by seeking treatment if and when we do get sick.

Or maybe we are just intimidated by the scope of the problem. We see the challenge of our declining life expectancy as too large, as beyond our capacity to correct.

If we continue to ignore, even accept, our collective poor health, it is in part because we have accepted changes in the past 30 years—such as growing income inequality—that have made our health worse. But these trends were not always on the rise, and our health was not always worse than our peer countries. As recently as 30 years ago, we were in the top half of the pack, when it came to health. If we have accepted our poor health, this acceptance is premature. It has lulled us into thinking our poor health is somehow inevitable, rather than a relatively recent development that can be linked to certain political policies, the reversal of which could change the trajectory of our health. Making this change means first talking honestly about where we are, and how we got here, so we can eventually get our health to where it should be.

## REFERENCES

Institute of Medicine, National Research Council. *US health in international perspective: shorter lives, poorer health*. Washington, DC: The National Academies Press; 2013.

Meredith S. US life expectancy is low and is now projected to be on par with Mexico by 2030. *CNBC*. February 22, 2017. https://www.cnbc.com/2017/02/22/us-life-expectancy-is-low-and-is-now-projected-to-be-on-par-with-mexico-by-2030.html Accessed September 17, 2019.

National Center for Health Statistics. Centers for Disease Control and Prevention Web site. https://www.cdc.gov/nchs/ Accessed September 17, 2019.

Newman K. US life expectancy falls as drug overdoses, suicides rise. *US News & World Report*. November 29, 2018. https://www.usnews.com/news/

healthiest-communities/articles/2018-11-29/us-life-expectancy-falls-as-drug-overdoses-suicides-rise Accessed September 17, 2019.

Spanish flu. History Web site. https://www.history.com/topics/world-war-i/1918-flu-pandemic Published October 12, 2010. Accessed September 17, 2019.

# 35

# NAMES MATTER IN THE OPIOID EPIDEMIC

Survey any number of media reports about drug use, and you will find mentions of "addicts" who use opioids. Casual conversations label individuals who use drugs as "junkies." We are accustomed to using language to distance ourselves from those with substance use problems, making sure we mark those who use drugs as "the other," as not like us.

Erving Goffman, one of the giants of 20th-century psychology, defined *stigma* as a "phenomenon whereby an individual with an attribute which is deeply discredited by his/her society is rejected as a result of the attribute. Stigma is a process by which the reaction of others spoils normal identity." That is exactly what we have done with drugs and the people who use them. We have used nouns to label those who use drugs so that they are discredited as a result of their behavior. This has consequences for their self-identity. Research carried out nearly two decades ago showed that persons who use drugs feel more marginalized because of their substance use than any other self-identification.

Little has changed in the ensuing years. The opioid epidemic now kills more people annually than the HIV epidemic at its worst, the firearm epidemic at its peak, or the most lethal year of motor vehicle accidents. And yet, despite near-saturation media

*Pained*. Michael D. Stein and Sandro Galea, Oxford University Press (2020). © Oxford University Press.
DOI: 10.1093/oso/9780197510384.001.0001

coverage of the problem, limited resources have been allocated toward tackling the epidemic. Surely part of the challenge is our ongoing stigmatization of those who use drugs. We have shown ourselves to be comfortable letting their problems remain their business, deluding ourselves into thinking their health is not intimately tied to our own. We can do this because we believe those who use drugs are "the other," and therefore could never be us. Continued use of marginalizing words in mass media reinforces this psychological distancing. Names have the power to separate.

The truth is, people who use drugs are not different from us, nor are they far away. The current epidemic has taught us that we all know someone who has developed a drug problem. In the face of this crisis, quibbling over words may seem like a distraction, a minor issue, but, in fact, using the right language to talk about drug use is a step toward ending this epidemic. It helps us remember drug use is not just a problem for "them," but for us all, and that only through compassion and collective effort can we effectively address the disease of addiction.

# REFERENCES

Bautista RE, Shapovalov D, Shoraka AR. Factors associated with increased felt stigma among individuals with epilepsy. *Seizure*. 2015; 30: 106–12. doi: 10.1016/j.seizure.2015.06.006

Minior T, Galea S, Stuber J, Ahern J, Ompad D. Racial differences in discrimination experiences and responses among minority substance users. *Ethnicity & Disease*. 2003; 13(4): 521–27.

Pivatova E, Stein MD. In their own words: Language preferences of individuals who use heroin. Addiction 2019; 114 (10): 1785–90.

# [ 36 ]

# PAIN DRAIN

We live in a country that is in pain. Approximately 20% of Americans suffer from chronic pain. Through lost work and often ineffective treatment, chronic pain costs us $600 billion annually, more than cancer and heart disease combined. The emotional and social toll is uncountable.

Pain exists at the crossroads of the two epidemics that have distinguished this decade: opioids and suicide. Pain and its mitigation were the rationale for the profligate (and deceptive) marketing of opioids between 1999 and 2014, when prescription pill sales quadrupled. That widespread misuse and addiction followed is, perhaps, not surprising. Physical pain is sometimes at the root of psychic pain, and isolation and despair can produce another form of suffering, leading to suicide.

What we know now is that pain starts as a symptom—associated, for example, with arthritis or neuropathy—and, for one in five Americans, this symptom becomes "chronic," that is, it lasts for weeks, or months, or even years. At some point during this period, the symptom becomes its own disease. Chronic pain has its own reliable neurobiology (which we are just beginning to understand) and its own brain activation signature—although it cannot be localized in any specific "pain area" like other sensory

*Pained.* Michael D. Stein and Sandro Galea, Oxford University Press (2020). © Oxford University Press. DOI: 10.1093/oso/9780197510384.001.0001

perceptions, such as smell or sight. Still, pain changes the brain's structure, its neuronal configurations.

Pain's significance in a person's life is highly individualized. The experience of chronic pain can be altered by mood, sleep quality, distraction, suggestion, or even anticipation of new pain. This implies that pain may be exacerbated by social conditions—by violence, by anxiety. Living in poverty, for example, increases the odds of living with chronic pain.

Pain is real; pain is also doubted and disputed. In our legal system, it is the subject of arguments over payment for disability claims and personal injury suits. The lack of an objective measure of pain means that someone who might deserve compensation misses out because she cannot "prove" her discomfort. Pain is always a subjective experience, but there is a race to make it more demonstrable—through brain scans, for example, and blood tests.

Pain makes us feel helpless. It makes us ruminate and catastrophize. Decreasing avoidable suffering is central to our sense of being healthy. To become and remain pain-free is a nearly universally shared life goal. Assessing and treating pain, recognizing the pain of others, coping with its presence, and limiting its ruinous effects without misusing opioids or taking one's own life remain central tests of our empathy and our efforts to promote health.

## REFERENCES

Dahlhamer J, Lucas J, Zelaya C, et al. Prevalence of chronic pain and high-impact chronic pain among adults—United States, 2016. *Morbidity and Mortality Weekly Report (MMWR)*. 2018; 67(36): 1001–6.

Niculescu AB, Le-Niculescu H, Levey DF, et al. Towards precision medicine for pain: diagnostic biomarkers and repurposed drugs. *Molecular Psychiatry*. 2019; 24(4): 501–22.

Opioid overdose. Centers for Disease Control and Prevention Web site. https://www.cdc.gov/drugoverdose/epidemic/index.html   Accessed September 17, 2019.

# VIOLENCE IS A PUBLIC HEALTH ISSUE

In the United States, nearly 20 people are physically abused by an intimate partner every minute. One in three women, and one in four men, are victims of some form of physical violence by an intimate partner at some point in their lives. Nearly 18,000 people died from homicide in the United States in 2017, with more than two thirds of those deaths due to firearms.

According to the *World Report on Violence and Health*, violence is "the intentional use of physical force or power . . . against oneself or against a group or community . . . that has a high likelihood of resulting in injury, death, psychological harm." Globally, nearly 4,000 people die due to violence every day, and about 100,000 are injured severely enough that they require medical attention. That is about 36 million people annually, or four times more people than die annually from cancer.

Even as rates of violence from several causes have declined, the persistent prevalence of violence in our daily lives, both domestically and globally, should give us pause. In theory, violence is eminently preventable. Decreasing violence should therefore be a top priority in our broader pursuit of disease prevention and improved health. Yet violence continues to injure and kill worldwide.

*Pained*. Michael D. Stein and Sandro Galea, Oxford University Press (2020). © Oxford University Press.
DOI: 10.1093/oso/9780197510384.001.0001

At the heart of our failure to prevent violence is the belief that violence is not a health issue. Overwhelmingly, we think of violence as a criminal justice problem, or a sociopolitical concern. This has resulted in our heavy-handed approach to incarceration, which has exacerbated racial divides in the United States and done little to prevent violence.

Yet violence *is* a public health problem, with consequences both individual and collective. Some individuals who experience violence die; those who do not will go on to bear a physical or mental health burden that can last a lifetime.

Because violence is a public health issue, solutions to violence must be rooted in a public health perspective. This means understanding how the context that shapes our health each day can raise the likelihood of violence, if we let it. We must work to improve this context, rather than simply punish offenders, if we are to create a world with less violence and better health.

## REFERENCES

Krug E, Dahlberg L, Mercy J, et al. *World report on violence and health.* Geneva: World Health Organization; 2002.

National Center for Health Statistics: assault or homicide. Centers for Disease Control and Prevention Web site. https://www.cdc.gov/nchs/fastats/homicide.htm Accessed September 17, 2019.

Scope of the problem: statistics. Rape, Abuse & Incest National Network Web site. https://www.rainn.org/statistics/scope-problem Accessed September 18, 2019.

Statistics. National Coalition Against Domestic Violence Web site. https://ncadv.org/statistics Accessed September 17, 2019.

Understanding and addressing violence against women. World Health Organization Web site. https://apps.who.int/iris/bitstream/handle/10665/77431/WHO_RHR_12.43_eng.pdf;jsessionid=00C2EDBCB4EDB5D0AD84BC4055125496?sequence=1 Accessed September 18, 2019.

# [ 38 ]

# MENTAL HEALTH
# AND MORTALITY

Mental illness contributes more to disability-adjusted life years than any other condition worldwide, with unipolar depression leading the way. And yet efforts to promote health continually deprioritize mental health. There are many reasons for this, starting with the historical stigma around mental illness and continuing with our limited understanding of the brain processes, at the cellular and molecular level, that underlie our behavior.

Then there is the sheer scope of deaths associated with mental health disorders. Most obvious are deaths due to suicide. There are about 1 million suicide deaths a year worldwide, or about one every 40 seconds, and suicide is the second leading cause of death among 15- to 29-year-olds globally. Far from the popular rendering of suicide as a problem only for wealthy nations, more than 75% of all suicides happen in low- and middle-income countries. Mental illness is the clearest driver of suicide.

But suicide is not the only form of mortality linked to mental health. Deaths caused by cigarette smoking, for example, are really deaths due to nicotine addiction; that is, 6 million deaths a year, or one every 5 seconds. And the more than 3 million deaths a year linked to alcohol stem from misuse of the substance—a mental health problem. Indeed, it is important to remember that any

*Pained.* Michael D. Stein and Sandro Galea, Oxford University Press (2020). © Oxford University Press. DOI: 10.1093/oso/9780197510384.001.0001

time we talk about substance use disorder, we are actually talking about mental health.

The consequences of mental illness are extensive. We must include them in any discussion of the health burden of noncommunicable disease. Only then will we give mental health the attention it deserves.

# REFERENCES

Alcohol. World Health Organization Web site. https://www.who.int/en/news-room/fact-sheets/detail/alcohol Accessed September 18, 2019.

Mental health: suicide data. World Health Organization Web site. https://www.who.int/mental_health/prevention/suicide/suicideprevent/en/ Accessed September 18, 2019.

Tobacco. World Health Organization Web site. https://www.who.int/en/news-room/fact-sheets/detail/tobacco Accessed September 18, 2019.

Whiteford HA, Degenhardt L, Rehm J, et al. Global burden of disease attributable to mental and substance use disorders: findings from the Global Burden of Disease Study 2010. *The Lancet*. 2013; 382(9904): 1575–86. doi: 10.1016/S0140-6736(13)61611-6

# 39

# THREE NOTES ON THE OPIOID CRISIS

We are in the midst of the greatest American health crisis of the century, an opioid epidemic that has now led to an astounding 500,000 deaths in the past two decades. There has been substantial attention devoted—appropriately—to this issue. However, there are three areas that receive far less attention than they should. One relates to the silent, concurrent increase in substance use that is occurring involving drugs other than opioids, the second relates to our perception of who is affected by opioids, and the third concerns our best hope of stemming this crisis.

First, while opioids have attracted most of the headlines, two other drugs are being misused in America at newly alarming rates, their rise paralleling that of opioids. These are cocaine and its prescription-based stimulant cousins, such as Adderall and Ritalin. The availability of cocaine has risen, and, with it, there has been a 60% rise in cocaine overdose deaths in the past 5 years. As with opioids, cocaine addiction is a chronic relapsing condition that requires repeated treatment interventions. But unlike treatments for opioids, which are effective at reducing deaths, treatments for cocaine have extremely modest effects. With fentanyl now getting mixed into cocaine batches, even occasional cocaine use has become notably lethal.

*Pained*. Michael D. Stein and Sandro Galea, Oxford University Press (2020). © Oxford University Press. DOI: 10.1093/oso/9780197510384.001.0001

With increases in prescriptions of attention-deficit/hyperactivity disorder (ADHD) medications—increases of over 50% in the past decade—there has been an accompanying increase in the nonmedical use of prescription stimulants. Stimulants are now the second most common drug misused on college campuses, after marijuana, with 15%–35% of college students having tried them recreationally—to study longer, concentrate better, get high, or lose weight—with ill effects on mood and sleep, and an increasing potential for addiction.

Then there is the issue of who is affected by opioids. This opioid tsunami has given us countless news stories about the toll on white, middle-class, suburban, and rural users. While there have indeed been dramatic increases in opioid deaths in these groups, the opioid-related deaths of black Americans have doubled in the past 15 years. In some states, blacks experience opioid-related deaths at higher rates than other racial or ethnic groups. We must remind ourselves this is not just a white epidemic.

Finally, because access to treatment for opioid addiction remains fragile, with national treatment rates low, we should keep in mind that Medicaid remains a key source of coverage for many people who use drugs. As we shore up a treatment system for opioid, cocaine, and stimulant misuse that has been woefully inadequate, threats to Medicaid's structure and funding need ongoing attention, or the consequences of drug use will continue to grow.

## REFERENCES

Benson K, Flory K, Humphreys KL, Lee SS. Misuse of stimulant medication among college students: a comprehensive review and meta-analysis. *Clinical Child and Family Psychology Review*. 2015; 18(1): 50–76. doi: 10.1007/s10567-014-0177-z

Chai G, Governale L, McMahon AW, Trinidad JP, Staffa J, Murphy D. Trends of outpatient prescription drug utilization in US children, 2002–2010. *Pediatrics*. 2012; 130(1): 23–31. doi: 10.1542/peds.2011-2879

Krawczyk N, Feder KA, Fingerhood MI, Saloner B. Racial and ethnic differences in opioid agonist treatment for opioid use disorder in a US national sample. *Drug and Alcohol Dependence*. 2017; 178: 512–18. doi: 10.1016/j.drugalcdep.2017.06.009

Rudd RA, Seth P, David F, Scholl L. Increases in drug and opioid-involved overdose deaths—United States, 2010–2015. *Morbidity and Mortality Weekly Report (MMWR)*. 2016; 65(50–51): 1445–52.

# 40

# INVEST IN HEALTH, NOT DEATH

We all die and, despite some fanciful ideas to the contrary, we will, as a species, continue to do so. Our daily routines tend to distract us from this fact. However, because death is inevitable, we need to think about how we can live healthy lives, without ignoring how they end.

Once we accept that we are going to die, how we spend our money and our time on health begins to shift. At core, we should aspire to die healthy. That means focusing our energy on creating a world that maximizes health right up until the moment we leave it, rather than one where we invest our resources into the last few months of life, ignoring the factors that keep us healthy all the years prior. This would represent a radical shift in how we think about our limited health investment dollars. Perhaps death can help focus our mind on living better, on the conditions that we need to create in order to generate health.

Of course, we should not neglect the experience of dying. We all wish to die with dignity, yet we do little, in advance, to influence the circumstances of our deaths. Two out of three Americans do not have advance directives that guide what treatments they receive if they are sick, and they cannot communicate the end-of-life care that they want. Engaging in a dialogue about how we manage the dying process can help us correct this oversight.

*Pained*. Michael D. Stein and Sandro Galea, Oxford University Press (2020). © Oxford University Press.
DOI: 10.1093/oso/9780197510384.001.0001

It is also important to remember those who are left. The dead leave behind the grieving, who can experience a burden of poor health that is directly linked to loss of their loved one. The sudden, unexpected death of a loved one is, for example, the largest contributor to posttraumatic stress disorder (PTSD) in populations. Death leaves behind lonely older adults, now socially isolated, placing them at higher risk of dying sooner. In this way, death creates a population health challenge for the living, one that is foreseeable and, perhaps, preventable.

Our squeamishness in talking about death is entirely natural. But it remains our collective role to elevate issues that influence the health of populations; death is one of those issues. Perhaps recognizing the inevitability of death can guide us toward ways in which we can live healthier, die with dignity, and ensure our loved ones are supported when we pass on.

## REFERENCES

Bell M. Why 5% of patients create 50% of health care costs. *Forbes*. January 10, 2013. https://www.forbes.com/sites/michaelbell/2013/01/10/why-5-of-patients-create-50-of-health-care-costs/#395b1a5528d7. Accessed September 17, 2019.

Can Google solve death? *Time*. September 30, 2013. http://content.time.com/time/covers/0,16641,20130930,00.html. Accessed September 17, 2019.

Keyes KM, Pratt C, Galea S, McLaughlin KA, Koenen KC, Shear MK. The burden of loss: Unexpected death of a loved one and psychiatric disorders across the life course in a national study. *American Journal of Psychiatry*. 2014; 171(8): 864–71.

Preidt R. 2 of 3 Americans don't have "advance directive" for end of life. *US News & World Report*. July 7, 2017. https://health.usnews.com/health-care/articles/2017-07-07/2-of-3-americans-dont-have-advance-directive-for-end-of-life. Accessed September 17, 2019.

# 41

# DIRECT-TO-DOCS OPIOID MARKETING

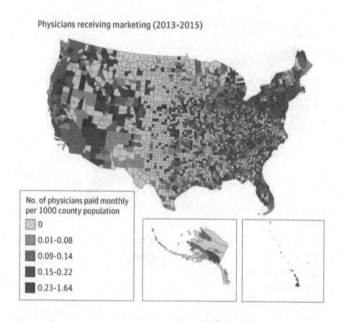

Physicians receiving marketing (2013-2015)

No. of physicians paid monthly
per 1000 county population
- 0
- 0.01-0.08
- 0.09-0.14
- 0.15-0.22
- 0.23-1.64

One factor that has fueled the current addiction epidemic is the pharmaceutical industry's direct-to-physician marketing of opioids. To promote new drugs, pharmaceutical companies often market their products to physicians by providing industry-sponsored meals, grants, and subsidies for continued medical

*Pained*. Michael D. Stein and Sandro Galea, Oxford University Press (2020). © Oxford University Press.
DOI: 10.1093/oso/9780197510384.001.0001

education and training. Physicians have also received fees for consulting or speaking publicly about opioid products, which sponsors bet could increase prescriptions among these doctors' peers.

A 2019 study sought to understand the relationship between mortality from opioid overdose and the pharmaceutical industry's direct marketing of opioids to physicians. The study analyzed the association between three factors in every US county: the amount of marketing payments pharmaceutical companies made to physicians, opioid prescribing rates, and the number of overdose deaths.

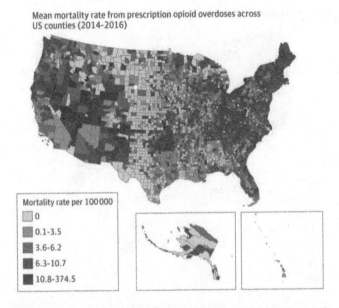

Mean mortality rate from prescription opioid overdoses across US counties (2014-2016)

Mortality rate per 100 000
- 0
- 0.1-3.5
- 3.6-6.2
- 6.3-10.7
- 10.8-374.5

Researchers found that direct marketing of opioids to physicians was associated with increased opioid prescribing rates and increased overdose mortality 1 year after marketing engagements. The first figure illustrates the number of physicians who received direct marketing between 2013 and 2015. The second figure highlights overdose mortality rate across the United States 1 year later (2014 to 2016). Higher prescribing rates are the link between opioid marketing to physicians and population mortality from overdoses.

The national response to the opioid epidemic has focused in part on reducing the number of opioids prescribed by physicians. Additionally, the Physician Payments Sunshine Act promotes financial transparency between pharmaceutical companies and health care providers. The Act requires any payments from companies to doctors be reported to the Centers for Medicaid and Medicare Services. States that have additional reporting requirements or limitations beyond those stipulated by the Physician Payments Sunshine Act include, as of this writing, Vermont, Massachusetts, Minnesota, Washington, DC, West Virginia, California, Connecticut, Louisiana, and Nevada.

By increasing regulation around pharmaceutical direct-to-physician marketing, and by making reports of pharmaceutical company payments to physicians available to the public, states have the potential to reduce overdose mortality.

# REFERENCES

Figures from Hadland SE, Rivera-Aguirre A, Marshall BDL, Cerdá M. Association of pharmaceutical industry marketing of opioid products with mortality from opioid-related overdoses. 2019; 2(1): e186007. doi: 10.1001/jamanetworkopen.2018.6007

Physicians and teaching hospitals. Centers for Medicare & Medicaid Services Web site. https://www.cms.gov/OpenPayments/Program-Participants/Physicians-and-Teaching-Hospitals/Physicians-and-Teaching-Hospitals.html Accessed September 19, 2019.

Reid L. The speakers' bureau system: a form of peer selling. *Open Medicine*. 2013; 7(2): e31–39.

Sullivan T. Physician Payments Sunshine Act: Review of individual state reporting requirements. *Policy & Medicine*. Last updated May 6, 2018. https://www.policymed.com/2014/04/physician-payments-sunshine-act-review-of-individual-state-reporting-requirements.html Accessed September 19, 2019.

Yeh JS, Franklin JM, Avorn J, Landon J, Kesselheim AS. Association of industry payments to physicians with the prescribing of brand-name statins in Massachusetts. *JAMA Internal Medicine*. 2016; 176(6): 763–68. doi: 10.1001/jamainternmed.2016.1709

# 42

# FIREARM LEGISLATION LINKED WITH FEWER FATAL POLICE SHOOTINGS

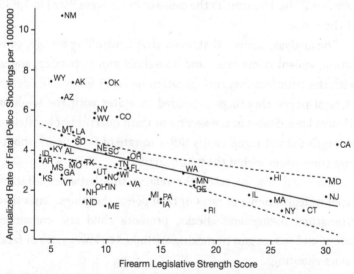

*Note.* Line represents regression line with 95% confidence interval (*P* < 0.001).
*Source.* Police shooting are from *The Guardian's* online database. The Counted and firearm legislative strength is form The Brady Center's legislative scorecards.

States with stricter firearm legislation have fewer fatal police shootings—defined as the rate of people killed by law enforcement agencies.

*Pained.* Michael D. Stein and Sandro Galea, Oxford University Press (2020). © Oxford University Press.
DOI: 10.1093/oso/9780197510384.001.0001

The authors of a 2017 study used two data sources to show this relationship. First, to determine the strength of state-level legislation, they used the Brady Center to Prevent Gun Violence's legislative scorecard for firearm laws. The scorecard highlights seven categories of laws, such as background checks, duty to retreat, and banning guns from public places. The higher the score, the stronger the firearm legislation is within that state.

Second, they used *The Counted*, an online database produced by *The Guardian*, to assess the number of fatal police shootings. This database uses news accounts, open-source reporting projects, and user submissions. A total of 2,021 fatal police encounters occurred in the United States between January 2015 and October 2016. Firearms as the cause of death were listed in 1,835 of the cases.

The analysis showed that, even after controlling for age, education, violent crime rates, and household gun ownership, states with the strongest firearm legislation had a 51% lower incidence of fatal police shootings compared to states with the weakest firearm laws. States in the second or third quartiles of legislative strength did not significantly differ in rate of fatal police shootings from states within the first quartile.

The study also assessed the relationship between different types of legislation and rates of fatal police shootings. Laws that strengthen background checks, promote child and consumer safety, and reduce gun trafficking are linked to lower rates of fatal police shootings.

The mechanisms at play, and the relative importance of individual types of law, are up for debate. However, the relationship demonstrated here is clear—stronger state-level firearm legislation is associated with lower rates of fatal police shootings.

# REFERENCES

Brady Center to Prevent Gun Violence Web site. https://www.bradyunited.
org Accessed September 19, 2019.

The Counted. *The Guardian*. https://www.theguardian.com/us-news/series/
counted-us-police-killings Accessed September 19, 2019.

Figure from Kivisto AJ, Ray B, Phalen PL. Firearm legislation and fatal police
shootings in the United States. *American Journal of Public Health*. 2017;
107(7): 1068–75. doi: 10.2105/AJPH.2017.303770

# THE FUNDAMENTALS

*We have created a country with health haves and health have-nots, with hundreds of millions of citizens whose health has been left behind. Who are these people? What are the challenges they face? And, crucially, what can we do to improve their health?*

# 43

# HOUSING AND
# THE PUBLIC'S HEALTH

Such since the early days of public health, housing has been recognized as a foundational determinant of health. In the 19th century, outbreaks of infectious diseases sparked interest in housing
reform as a means of addressing poor sanitation, crowding, and
inadequate ventilation. Over 150 years later, a report from the
World Health Organization (WHO) commission on the social
determinants of health returned to the concept of "safe housing"
as key to the health of populations.

There are ample data linking poor housing conditions to a
broad range of infectious diseases, chronic diseases, injuries,
childhood development and nutrition issues, and mental health
concerns. For example, substandard housing conditions such as
poor ventilation, pest infestation, and water leaks are directly
associated with the development and exacerbation of respiratory
diseases, such as asthma. There are about 24 million Americans
with asthma, and it is the most common chronic disease among
children worldwide. About 40% of diagnosed childhood asthma is
attributed to exposures at home.

The burden of poor housing is not distributed evenly across
populations. Families with fewer resources are likelier to live in
unhealthy homes, and they are less likely to be able to improve

*Pained*. Michael D. Stein and Sandro Galea, Oxford University Press (2020). © Oxford University Press.
DOI: 10.1093/oso/9780197510384.001.0001

the condition of their living situations. In addition, high housing costs often put families and individuals in the position of having to trade between healthy housing and other basic necessities, such as food or medication.

The forces of income segregation and racial/ethnic segregation have an enormous effect on housing suitability and health. In large metropolitan areas, the percentage of families living in "poor" or "rich" neighborhoods increased from 15% in 1970 to 34% in 2012. Moreover, disparities in housing based on racial background are substantial. Approximately 7.5% of non-Hispanic blacks and 2.8% of whites live in substandard housing. Those living in poor and dangerous housing are disproportionally low-income and people of color; it is not surprising, then, that the rate of asthma in black children is nearly two times higher than the rate of asthma in white children.

Structural forces perpetuate housing inequities. Landlords and real estate agents have contributed to racial/ethnic segregation by blocking minorities from moving to predominately white neighborhoods, which often leads to the exclusion of minorities from high-quality housing, schools, and other public services. Further, predominantly minority communities receive less investment from lenders to improve housing quality and neighborhood environments. Improving housing must also mean improving housing equity, so that all can access the benefits of having a safe, healthy place to live.

## REFERENCES

Asher I, Pearce N. Global burden of asthma among children. *The International Journal of Tuberculosis and Lung Disease*. 2014; 18(11): 1269–78. doi: 10.5588/ijtld.14.0170

Children's environmental health disparities: black and African American children and asthma. United States Environmental Protection Agency Web site. https://www.epa.gov/sites/production/files/2014-05/documents/hd_aa_asthma.pdf Accessed September 19, 2019.

Commission on Social Determinants of Health. *Closing the gap in a generation: health equity through action on the social determinants of health. Final Report of the Commission on Social Determinants of Health*. Geneva: World Health Organization; 2008.

Jacobs DE. Environmental health disparities in housing. *American Journal of Public Health*. 2011; 101(Suppl 1): S115–S122. doi: 10.2105/AJPH.2010.300058

Krieger J, Higgins DL. Housing and health: time again for public health action. *American Journal of Public Health*. 2002; 92(5): 758–68.

Lanphear BP, Aligne CA, Auinger P, Weitzman M, Byrd RS. Residential exposures associated with asthma in US children. *Pediatrics*. 2001; 107(3): 505–11.

Lanphear BP, Kahn RS, Berger O, Auinger P, Bortnick SM, Nahhas RW. Contribution of residential exposures to asthma in us children and adolescents. *Pediatrics*. 2001; 107(6): E98.

Learn how to control asthma. Centers for Disease Control and Prevention Web site. https://www.cdc.gov/asthma/faqs.htm Accessed September 19, 2019.

National Center for Health Statistics: Asthma. Centers for Disease Control and Prevention Web site. https://www.cdc.gov/nchs/fastats/asthma.htm Accessed September 19, 2019.

Reardon SF, Bischoff K. The continuing increase in income segregation, 2007–2012. Stanford Center for Education Policy Analysis Web site. https://cepa.stanford.edu/sites/default/files/the%20continuing%20increase%20in%20income%20segregation%20march2016.pdf Accessed September 19, 2019.

Turner MA, et al. Housing discrimination against racial and ethnic minorities 2012: full report. HUD USER Web site. https://www.huduser.gov/portal/Publications/pdf/HUD-514_HDS2012.pdf Accessed September 19, 2019.

# 44

# FOOD JUSTICE

One in six people in the United States experiences food insecurity. Forty-two million low-income and working-class Americans— most of whom are elderly, disabled, or children—use Supplemental Nutrition Assistance Program (SNAP) benefits to buy groceries. That is, they don't earn enough to feed themselves consistently. Food insecurity has dramatic effects on the health of children and the elderly in particular, influencing educational progress, family stress, and nutritional deficiencies. Yet, as millions of Americans remain food insecure, we throw away 40% of our food every day. That's 400 pounds per person, per year.

The largest source of this waste is the food we buy and bring home; 70% of all food discarded in our homes is edible. Restaurants are second in waste generation. Grocery stores, third in line, are a major source of usable, donatable goods, like fruits, vegetables, meat, and other nutritious foods. A fifth of agricultural water use and 18% of farm fertilizer is spent on food that is lost. Wasted food generates pollution equivalent to 37 million cars (2.6% of greenhouse emissions) through methane released from our land-fills. We waste 50% more food than we did 50 years ago.

If we could recover and redistribute one third of the food we waste, we could end food insecurity. Other countries are already

*Pained.* Michael D. Stein and Sandro Galea, Oxford University Press (2020). © Oxford University Press.
DOI: 10.1093/oso/9780197510384.001.0001

moving in this direction. In France, a 2016 law banned grocery stores from throwing away edible food. Giving food to churches or food banks is no longer just an act of good will there; it is becoming mandatory, with stores fined for not donating. Italy, for its part, has incentivized waste reduction, with the government funding active research on packing food to prevent spoilage and extend shelf life.

We may be starting to take similar steps in the United States. The 2018 Farm Bill supports food waste reduction plans in 10 states, creates a new Food Loss and Waste Liaison position within the US Department of Agriculture, and, following the European example, promotes the expansion of liability protections for food donations. In the private sector, there has been a rush of money into food waste reduction start-ups.

Reducing food waste creates economic, environmental, and public health benefits, as well as jobs, climate change deceleration, and hunger relief. Wasting food is a luxury, which we, increasingly, cannot afford. We must do our best to ensure we waste nothing, so that none go hungry.

## REFERENCES

2018 US Food Waste Investment Report. ReFED Web site. https://www.refed.com/download#food-waste-investment-report    Accessed September 19, 2019.

Congress's conference report solidifies Farm Bill support for major food waste reduction measures. Farm Bill Law Enterprise Web site (Cross-posted from the Center for Health Law and Policy Innovation Blog). http://www.farmbilllaw.org/2018/12/12/food_waste_conference/ Accessed September 19, 2019.

Hall KD, Guo J, Dore M, Chow CC. The progressive increase of food waste in America and its environmental impact. *PLOS One*. 2009; 4(11): e7940. doi: 10.1371/journal.pone.0007940

Heller MC, Keoleian GA. Greenhouse gas emission estimates of US dietary choices and food loss. *Journal of Industrial Ecology*. 2014; 19(3): 391–401.

Save the Food Web site. https://savethefood.com Accessed September 19, 2019.

# 45

# GUNS AND SUICIDE

Suicide is one of the very few causes of death that have remained stubbornly steady over nearly the past century. A 2018 CDC report showed that suicide rates have risen about 30% in the United States since 1999. The report revealed an increase in suicide among all sexes, racial/ethnic groups, and ages. In 2016 there were nearly 45,000 suicides in the United States; suicide is now the tenth leading cause of death in the country.

Suicidologists have long noted that there is no single cause of suicide. Although individuals with medical illness and substance use history are at greater risk of suicide, fully half of all individuals who commit suicide have no known history of a mental health diagnosis. Reflecting this, the National Strategy for Suicide Prevention calls for a broad range of approaches at the individual, family, and community level. Such approaches will make a difference over time. However, there is something we can do, right now, to reduce suicides. What if we focused on preventing suicide by limiting the means to commit suicide?

There is precedent for this. South Korea has long had suicide rates higher than other high-income countries. In the 2006–2010 time period, suicide by pesticides accounted for more than a fifth of all suicides in the country. Then South Korea banned the sale of

*Pained.* Michael D. Stein and Sandro Galea, Oxford University Press (2020). © Oxford University Press.
DOI: 10.1093/oso/9780197510384.001.0001

paraquat—the leading pesticide—in 2012. This was followed by an immediate decline in suicide rates across all groups.

The success of such an effort rests on a simple observation: close to half of all suicides are acts of impulse, decided with an hour, if not a few minutes, before the suicide itself. This means that having access to lethal means matters enormously. And lethality varies between means. The likelihood of a successful suicide by drug overdose is less than 10%; the likelihood of successful suicide by gun is more than 90%. That means, with guns around, the suicidal impulse is much more likely to end in the act's completion.

Is it surprising, then, given how many guns we have in the country, that firearms account for about half of all suicides in the United States—more than 22,000 deaths in 2016. There are plenty of reasons for gun safety measures in this country. Surely as we discuss suicide, measures to limit the role of guns should be part of the national conversation.

## REFERENCES

Follman M. No, mental illness is not the main cause of mass shootings in America. *Mother Jones*. October 27, 2015. https://www.motherjones.com/crime-justice/2015/10/mental-health-gun-laws-washington-post-poll/ Accessed September 20, 2019.

Miller M, Hemenway D. Guns and suicide in the United States. *The New England Journal of Medicine*. 2008; 359(10): 989–91. doi: 10.1056/NEJMp0805923

National Center for Health Statistics: suicide and self-inflicted injury. Centers for Disease Control and Prevention Web site. https://www.cdc.gov/nchs/fastats/suicide.htm Accessed September 20, 2019.

Stone DM, Simon TR, Fowler KA, et al. Vital signs: trends in state suicide rates—United States, 1999–2016 and circumstances contributing to suicide—27 states, 2015. *Morbidity and Mortality Weekly Report (MMWR)*. 2018; 67(22): 617–24.

*World health statistics 2017: monitoring health for the SDGs, sustainable development goals*. Geneva: World Health Organization; 2017.

# 46

# THE SMOKING GAP

Four in 10 American adults smoked cigarettes in 1965; only 15% smoke today. That's an impressive public health success, but it should not be the end of the story. There remain 40 million smokers in the United States who will suffer cancer and cardiovascular consequences from the dozens of harmful chemicals in tobacco products for decades to come, at a cost of $300 billion per year.

Fifty years ago, smoking prevalence for all education groups was clustered at that 40%–45% mark. Five decades later, 6.5% of college-educated individuals continue to smoke, while the prevalence is more than triple that among those with a high school education or less (23.1%). These smokers tend to be disadvantaged socially and economically, and bear the majority of morbidity and premature mortality. Education also seems to matter.

So we have lowered smoking overall, and in the process, we have created a smoking gap between those who are well educated and those who are less educated, between those with higher and lower incomes.

And the smoking gap is not restricted only to socioeconomic status. Geography is also at play. "Tobacco Nation," a swath across the American Southeast where 700 million pounds of tobacco are harvested annually, and rates of smoking remain higher than elsewhere, suggests that policy, culture, and the persistent influence

*Pained.* Michael D. Stein and Sandro Galea, Oxford University Press (2020). © Oxford University Press.
DOI: 10.1093/oso/9780197510384.001.0001

of the tobacco industry in this region has shaped who smokes and who does not in the United States. At the county level, rural dwellers have higher rates of cigarette use, which may or may not result from intentional industry targeting. Workplace smoking bans will not lead to cessation among people who work outdoors or who are unemployed, two conditions notable in rural areas.

Other studies have documented the high tobacco retailer density in neighborhoods with larger proportions of African Americans, the ethnic group with the highest smoking prevalence. This causal relationship may work in both directions: more retailers sell tobacco because there are more tobacco users, and current smokers smoke more tobacco because there is heightened exposure to these tobacco retail environments.

What do we learn from the smoking gap?

First, this is part of a pattern which we observe in health. Efforts to fix the immediate health behavior (in this case smoking) fall short when we do not deal with the underlying problem— often one of social or economic disadvantage. This has been well documented in medical sociology and is called the fundamental cause hypothesis.

Second, innovative interventions, implemented at the national, state, community, and local levels and focused on disadvantaged groups, provide the best chance to lower the smoking rate further. But it will take a series of such actions, based on evidence. These include setting minimum pricing policies across states; strategic partnerships with the 2-1-1 phone system whose callers are disproportionally low income, unemployed, and/or uninsured; reducing sales of untaxed or low-tax cigarettes; social branding interventions that target young adults and look to prevent smoking initiation; supporting the ban on smoking in public housing; and expanding care access to smoking-cessation counseling and medication benefits via Medicaid expansion. Electronic cigarettes represent another avenue to improve the health of smokers, and there is now evidence that e-cigarette use can lead to smoking cessation. There are certainly other approaches and policies worthy of consideration beyond this list.

Reducing the smoking rate to below 15% will be particularly challenging. But we know the best public health approach will need both to tackle the foundational problems that shape our health and target the populations at greatest risk.

## REFERENCES

Drope J, Liber AC, Cahn Z, et al. Who's still smoking? Disparities in adult cigarette smoking prevalence in the United States. *CA: A Cancer Journal for Clinicians.* 2018; 68(2): 106–15. doi: 10.3322/caac.21444

Dwyer-Lindgren L, Mokdad AH, Srebotnjak T, Flaxman AD, Hansen GM, Murray CJ. Cigarette smoking prevalence in US counties: 1996–2012. *Population Health Metrics.* 2014; 12(1): 5. doi: 10.1186/1478-7954-12-5

Levy DT, Huang AT, Havumaki JS, Meza R. The role of public policies in reducing smoking prevalence: results from the Michigan SimSmoke tobacco policy simulation model. *Cancer Causes & Control.* 2016; 27(5): 615–25. doi: 10.1007/s10552-016-0735-4

Smoking and tobacco use: economic trends in tobacco. Centers for Disease Control and Prevention Web site. https://www.cdc.gov/tobacco/data_statistics/fact_sheets/economics/econ_facts/index.htm Accessed September 20, 2019.

Weaver SR, Huang J, Pechacek TF, Heath JW, Ashley DL, Eriksen MP. Are electronic nicotine delivery systems helping cigarette smokers quit? Evidence from a prospective cohort study of US adult smokers, 2015–2016. *PLOS One.* 2018; 13(7): e0198047. doi: 10.1371/journal.pone.0198047

# 47

# MAYBE THE END OF HIV

For 40 years, HIV has been our most politically charged illness and a defining health challenge of our time. Our recollection of these decades contains visceral images of Kaposi's sarcoma, a quilt covering the National Mall, bodies of Giacometti emaciation, of Silence=Death written under overpasses, and of fake blood thrown on politicians. HIV has been a disease of private hiding and public protest. It has been the disease of demands: for civil rights, for medical rights, for open and shared science, for enhanced and coordinated funding. HIV and its trail of discontent has driven the study of health disparities and animated the work of global health.

At the same time, the world of HIV care over the last two decades has seen a great, almost miraculous, revolution. Today, a 35-year-old who was HIV-infected in 2018 and takes her daily medication adherently has the life expectancy of a 35-year-old without HIV infection. Monthly injections of long-acting HIV drugs look to be as good as daily pills at suppressing the virus, creating easier treatment. Medication to prophylactically prevent infection is 95% effective. Recent reports of two persons "cured" of HIV have created hope and impatience.

Despite these stunning advances, disparities in detection and care characterize the disease. More than half of new HIV cases in

*Pained*. Michael D. Stein and Sandro Galea, Oxford University Press (2020). © Oxford University Press.
DOI: 10.1093/oso/9780197510384.001.0001

the United States today occur in seven, mostly southern, states, in 48, mostly rural, counties. In these states, nearly half of the infected don't know they are infected and, therefore, are at risk of spreading the disease. Those who don't know their HIV status or are not receiving anti-viral treatment are connected to 81% of new infections. The epidemic has shifted to groups that are hard to test, hard to get started on preventive care, hard to keep on daily medication—persons who inject stimulants, men on the down-low, the mentally ill, the homeless, the rural poor with no health insurance. Lack of information, lack of trust of providers, unfamiliarity with services, and refusals of testing and treatment due to social rejection and privacy concerns make the delivery of care more challenging for these groups. Even among persons enrolled in AIDS clinical trials who have found their way to cutting-edge medical treatment, blacks and Hispanics have poorer outcomes.

The challenges that characterize HIV transmission in the United States will be hard to overcome. There will be upticks along the way, as other sexually transmitted infections rise and needle exchange programs remain outside the law or close up shop. And plans from government agencies to allow private Medicare plans not to cover certain drugs run directly counter to the goal of HIV elimination. Reaching an end to this disease will require new attention to health systems and social stigma, to geography, to housing and outreach, to the long work of public health.

## REFERENCES

Bhagwat P, Kapadia SN, Ribaudo HJ, Gulick RM, Currier JS. Racial disparities in virologic failure and tolerability during firstline HIV antiretroviral therapy. *Open Forum Infectious Diseases*. 2019; 6(2): ofz022. doi: 10.1093/ofid/ofz022

HIV in the United States by region. Centers for Disease Control and Prevention Web site. https://www.cdc.gov/hiv/statistics/overview/geographicdistribution.html Accessed September 20, 2019.

KHN morning briefing: Trump's budget contains $291 million funding boost for domestic HIV goals, but also cuts global aid to fight epidemic. *Kaiser Health News*. March 12, 2019. https://khn.org/morning-breakout/trumps-budget-contains-291-million-funding-boost-for-domestic-hiv-goals-but-also-cuts-global-aid-to-fight-epidemic/ Accessed September 20, 2019.

Mandavilli A. HIV is reported cured in a second patient, a milestone in the global AIDS epidemic. *The New York Times*. March 4, 2019. https://www.nytimes.com/2019/03/04/health/aids-cure-london-patient.html Accessed September 20, 2019.

# 48

# HOMELESSNESS

Homelessness is a brutal, demoralizing experience. Every day more than 550,000 Americans experience the difficult search for shelter, food, clothing, a place to wash, a place to go to the bathroom. Even those who find their way to shelters have three times the age-adjusted risk of dying compared to the general population. Those who go unsheltered, the so-called rough sleepers, have 10 times the mortality.

Homelessness has the power to move us to action like few other issues. Unfortunately, our efforts to tackle homelessness have fallen short. Historically, making housing contingent on sobriety and employment—forcing those who did not meet these marks to fall away and become chronically homeless—has imperiled millions. Encouragingly, Housing First—a program that provides housing and support services without requiring employment or pretreatment for mental health conditions and substance use disorders—has started to gain traction. The program has led to improvements in housing stability, reduced hospitalizations and use of emergency departments, and improved quality of life.

Making housing more permanent and affordable is an essential first step, if dual-edged. Moving the urban homeless from

*Pained.* Michael D. Stein and Sandro Galea, Oxford University Press (2020). © Oxford University Press.
DOI: 10.1093/oso/9780197510384.001.0001

their current situation offers protection, but also isolation from the little help and friendship known to these individuals, especially those with mental illness or disability. Still, rapid rehousing availability for those in need is critical.

Adding to this challenge, over 8 million more Americans are just one step away from homelessness. And unlike the homeless, they are often invisible. The number of renters with very low income, who use half of it for housing and receive no government assistance, has grown 25% in the past decade. Many become homeless through temporary personal or financial crises, and 40% of people experiencing homelessness are families with children. Preventing homelessness in these lower income households requires the creation of a living wage (impossible at $7.25 an hour, the current federal figure). But prevention is also about identifying risk and providing supportive services when an individual or family is on the brink.

About one in three homeless persons is a veteran, up from one in ten only a decade ago. The Department of Veterans Affairs has noted that ending homelessness requires two ingredients: individual planning and available housing stock. Even if homelessness cannot be fully prevented, it can be responded to with immediacy, resources, and an attitude that no one should stay on the street or in a shelter for long. A community with the support of state and federal government funding that offers collaborative programming and care can do what is needed.

Doing everything within our power to minimize homelessness is a matter of health equity. Efforts to address homelessness have made slow progress, but we should resist mission fatigue. Homelessness is a public health threat and a national disgrace. We must do all we can to end it.

# REFERENCES

National homeless rates decline, but severe housing cost burdens rise. National Low Income Housing Coalition Web site. https://nlihc. org/resource/national-homeless-rates-decline-severe-housing-cost-burdens-rise Published August 30, 2019. Accessed September 20, 2019.

New partnership aims to end chronic homelessness in 15 communities. Kaiser Permanente Web site. https://about.kaiserpermanente.org/ our-story/news/announcements/new-kaiser-permanente-partnership-aims-to-end-chronic-homelessne. Accessed September 20, 2019.

Palepu A, Patterson ML, Moniruzzaman A, Frankish CJ, Somers J. Housing First improves residential stability in homeless adults with concurrent substance dependence and mental disorders. *American Journal of Public Health*. 2013; 103(Suppl 2): e30–36. doi: 10.2105/AJPH.2013.301628

Roncarati JS, Baggett TP, O'Connell JJ, et al. Mortality among unsheltered homeless adults in Boston, Massachusetts, 2000–2009. *JAMA Internal Medicine*. 2018; 178(9): 1242–48. doi: 10.1001/ jamainternmed.2018.2924

# [ 49 ]

# DOCUMENTING DELAYS
# IN EMS WAIT TIMES

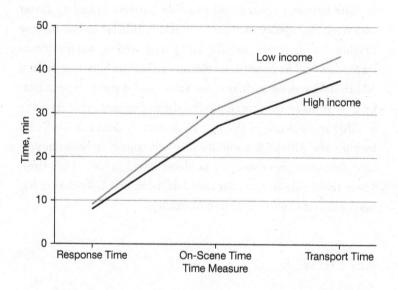

How long do you think it takes for an ambulance to respond
to a 9-1-1 call and get a patient to a hospital? In a 2018 study,
researchers assessed 63,000 cardiac arrest emergency medical services (EMS) encounters to determine whether ambulance
response times were longer in low-income versus high-income
urban zip codes. The graph displays three measures, comparing
low-income and high-income neighborhoods in (1) the time in

*Pained*. Michael D. Stein and Sandro Galea, Oxford University Press (2020). © Oxford University Press.
DOI: 10.1093/oso/9780197510384.001.0001

minutes between EMS dispatch to arrival at the patient's location (Response Time), (2) the time between EMS arrival and departure (On-Scene Time), and (3) the time between scene departure and arrival at the destination hospital (Transport Time).

The total EMS time (Response + On-Scene + Transport) for low-income communities was 3.8 minutes (10%) longer than in high-income neighborhoods. The gap in time between the two areas is largely attributable to On-Scene Time, which was 2.8 minutes (15%) longer in low-income zip codes. The authors do not give insight as to why on-scene time has the biggest difference in time between groups, but possible barriers impeding faster care from emergency medical technicians (EMTs) in low-income neighborhoods might include congested streets, narrow doorways, and buildings without elevators. The authors cite several additional barriers, such as scene safety and distance from a hospital, that may have contributed to the differences in total time.

This study is one of the first to document delays in EMS care by zip code. Although a minute may not appear to be an important difference, survival may be determined in this short time. The authors note that cardiac care delayed by just 1–4 minutes has been associated with increased mortality.

## REFERENCE

Figure from Hsia RY, Huang D, Mann NC, et al. A US national study of the association between income and ambulance response time in cardiac arrest. *JAMA Network Open*. 2018; 1(7): e185202. doi: 10.1001/jamanetworkopen.2018.5202

# 50

# PARTICULAR PARTICULATES

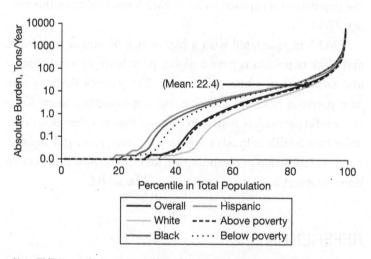

*Note.* PM2.5 = particulate matter of 2.5 micrometers in diameter or less. Burden scale (y-axis) is displayed logarithmatically. Poverty level determined by the US Censes Bureau in 2013.

Racially or ethnically marginalized and poor communities in the United States are likelier to be situated near landfills and pollution-producing industrial sites than majority white, affluent communities.

These facilities emit harmful air particulates that impact lung and heart health. Particulate matter (PM) in the air is a combination of solid and liquid pollutants. In general, the smaller the particles, the more harmful they are to health. A 2018 report offers

*Pained.* Michael D. Stein and Sandro Galea, Oxford University Press (2020). © Oxford University Press.
DOI: 10.1093/oso/9780197510384.001.0001

findings on the health impacts of disparate exposure to PM2.5, or particulate matter smaller than 2.5 micrometers in diameter.

The figure depicts the distribution of the PM2.5 burden, or the average tons of PM2.5 emitted per year at close proximity, by race, ethnicity, and poverty status. Hispanic and black Americans tend to have a higher PM2.5 burden than their white counterparts. Those below the federal poverty line experience more exposure to PM2.5 than those with higher incomes. Fifteen percent of the population is exposed to more PM2.5 per year than the average 22.4 tons.

PM2.5 is associated with a higher risk of illness and death, and black populations have a higher prevalence of heart disease and asthma than white populations. The report's findings confirm previous research documenting disproportionate exposure to harmful particulate matter in communities of color. These data show how health is inextricably tied to place, race, and the economic composition of communities. Identifying how these conditions intersect is key to creating a healthier world.

## REFERENCE

Figure from Mikati I, Benson AF, Luben TJ, Sacks JD, Richmond-Bryant J. Disparities in distribution of particulate matter emission sources by race and poverty status. *American Journal of Public Health*. 2018; 108(4): 480–85. doi: 10.2105/AJPH.2017.304297. Reproduced with permission.

# WILL TECHNOLOGY SAVE US?

*So much is written about health, and, in the past few years, much of this writing has been about the promise of technology, about how the newest app or social media platform is going to result in a health revolution. But will it? Is technology really the panacea it is often promoted to be? Will technology help us at all? How should we think about the role of technology in advancing health?*

# 51

# SHOULD BLACK BOXES BE WELCOME IN MEDICINE?

It has become an article of faith that technology will improve the practice of medicine in coming decades. Medicine enthusiastically embraces novel technical approaches that may improve patient care. But what if those technical approaches bring greater scrutiny to clinical work? What if they cast a harsh light on work that medicine typically does behind closed doors?

Such questions emerge as efforts grow to introduce "black boxes" to surgery.

When an airplane goes down, there is an urgent search for the plane's black box. The black box contains both the audio recording of all cockpit discussion, as well as a recording of flight instrument readings. These two flight recorders are required by international regulation and together offer the best possibility of learning what happened in the minutes preceding any aviation accident or incident.

A version of this kind of recording technology—which captures medical conversation and physiological parameters, allowing for postsurgery analysis—is starting to make its way into the world of medicine. Early reports suggest that intraoperative error events are far more frequent than previously noted, and a high number of operating room distractions inform these mistakes.

*Pained.* Michael D. Stein and Sandro Galea, Oxford University Press (2020). © Oxford University Press.
DOI: 10.1093/oso/9780197510384.001.0001

Black box recording devices would bring a new transparency to what actually happened during adverse events, allowing us to improve our surgical procedures.

But the operating room is a sacred space. Its sterilized choreography and chatter have never before been scrutinized in this way. The new technology raises important questions. Will surgeons (and other health professionals) be put in malpractice jeopardy by such new information? Will patients and their families become more likely to sue? Will more information undermine patient trust?

Surgical safety depends on team dynamics and communications, technical issues, and alertness and rapid response to a patient's trouble. Will constant surveillance produce a different kind of accountability and therefore a different level of stress? Will surgical staff be likelier to speak up when they see something amiss?

These questions will require sober assessment. But, at heart, we are an information culture, and medicine aspires to create a culture of continual improvement. We can imagine black box technology entering medicine widely over the next years, moving beyond surgical suites and into delivery rooms where maternal mortality is rising, and where we might study what goes wrong, identify solutions, and share lessons learned.

## REFERENCES

Jung JJ, Jüni P, Lebovic G, Grantcharov T. First-year analysis of the operating room black box study. *Annals of Surgery*. 2018. doi: 10.1097/SLA.0000000000002863

MacDorman MF, Declercq E, Cabral H, Morton C. Is the United States maternal mortality rate increasing? Disentangling trends from measurement issues. *Obstetrics & Gynecology*. 2016; 128(3): 447–55. doi: 10.1097/AOG.0000000000001556

# 52

# THE NEW ELDERLY
# SURVEILLANCE STATE

Millions of older adults will develop dementia over the coming decades. The middle-agers who assume responsibility for this older generation face a looming concern: how can we keep our parents safe and at home? Can technology help make this possible?

If media commentary on this subject is to be believed, the Internet of Things will carry part of the load of caring for our elders. New, in-home smart systems will reduce caregiver stress through electronic surveillance, allowing doctors to get real-time insights into the health of our loved ones, improving their quality of life.

Teams of clinical, economic, security, and technical experts are now at work on a new form of "assisted living." The model patient will have, in her home, passive environmental sensors (allowing, for example, the stove to turn itself off), medical devices, wearable technologies, and interactive apps connected to her body and bed, floor and door frames, collecting a fast-moving stream of data. Such "living labs" are already deployed and being evaluated. These new "trusted patient homes" will require a new kind of workforce of health care practitioners, not only persons who can read the new dashboards, but also technicians who can maintain the sensors. But will these new, technologically sophisticated

*Pained*. Michael D. Stein and Sandro Galea, Oxford University Press (2020). © Oxford University Press.
DOI: 10.1093/oso/9780197510384.001.0001

homes really tackle the core problems of aging and dementia? Yes, they will bring us more data. Yes, we might better understand the physiological patterns of persons living with dementia at scale. But can we really improve the lives of our elders with dementia, and their families, with easy-to-follow audio instructions piped in over speakers? Will a daughter feel safe leaving her mother alone at home in this surveilled new world?

Technology by itself will not be the full solution. Somewhere we have to figure out the role that old-fashioned social networks—humans checking in on humans—will play, and how technology can help augment, not replace, the role that caregivers play in maximizing quality of life for those who can no longer care for themselves. This will require a serious examination of the role of work and obligation, borne by those in middle age, and how this can fit in with the increasing responsibilities they will inevitably bear, as the population ages.

# [ 53 ]

# GOOD APP HUNTING

Public health and medicine are in a moment of digital euphoria. We have convinced ourselves that mhealth (mobile phone) technologies will improve the health of millions. After all, there are 6 billion smartphones out there, and more than 300,000 stand-alone health apps on the market, ready to be uploaded. Suddenly, the promise of using this technology to motivate behavior change—to reduce highly prevalent conditions like obesity, diabetes, anxiety, and insomnia—is scalable. But as behavioral health facilitators, will phone apps work? And how will we know if they do?

Health apps primarily perform three functions: they monitor, measure, and manage. The first generation of apps were largely about self-monitoring. These "do it yourself" kinds of apps had users record and consider their own data—food ingested, mood, glucose levels—and offered these users opportunities to modify their behavior. Next came measuring, quantifying apps, which soon became sensor-based, including recordings of heart rate, steps walked, sleep stages, and food labels. Such sensors limited manual input and offered novel "health" markers to monitor. We have now entered the era of the "prescribable" app—an app for the treatment of managing conditions anytime, anywhere. Some of these apps have even been recommended by health providers.

*Pained.* Michael D. Stein and Sandro Galea, Oxford University Press (2020). © Oxford University Press.
DOI: 10.1093/oso/9780197510384.001.0001

The most commonly trialed apps are those that are designed to address conditions with the largest global health burden: diabetes, mental health, and obesity. But of all the health apps on the market, only a few dozen have ever been tested using randomized trials. And these trials, as with most new treatments, involved few participants, assessed for short periods of time, and, in general, were poorly designed, performed, and analyzed. This should not be a surprise; funding sources for app development and testing are rare—a full-scale clinical trial can be long and expensive, and risks a negative result. Waiting for the demonstration of positive benefits is not yet the modus operandi of this new field.

In the digital world, faulty anecdotes of health success can go viral. We need a means for efficacy assessment and a reliable source of quality information—a Consumer Reports for health-related apps—and a recognized national organization that can evaluate and decide which are useful and safe. Even a modestly effective app, if available to millions of users, could have an enormous impact on the public's health. But the search for app evidence is challenging and takes time—a commodity of which few of us, in the digital age, have enough.

## REFERENCES

Byambasuren O, Sanders S, Beller E, Glasziou P. Prescribable mHealth apps identified from an overview of systematic reviews. *NPJ Digital Medicine*. 2018. doi: 10.1038/s41746-018-0021-9

Yardley L, Choudhury T, Patrick K, Michie S. Current issues and future directions for research into digital behavior change interventions. *American Journal of Preventive Medicine*. 2016; 51(5): 814–15. doi: 10.1016/j.amepre.2016.07.019.

# 54

# IN SOCIAL MEDIA WE TRUST

We have grown accustomed to social media reading our thoughts. One day, we are using Facebook to exchange notes about an upcoming wedding invitation, and, the next day, Facebook ads highlight discounts on potential wedding gifts. We post photos of a new item of clothing on Instagram, and we are soon receiving ads from the newest crop of design stars.

Of course, our social media accounts are not reading our thoughts—they are reading our photos, shopping patterns, and the words we write in our emails and posts. We have come to think of this type of targeted advertising as unremarkable, even as, in recent years, we have become more aware of the potential havoc such micro-targeting can wreak on our democratic process.

But what if this micro-targeting, instead of being only a force to generate consumer interest, were also a force for health? What if it offered a means of ameliorating a key public health problem, like Americans' growing suicide rate?

Let's say a hypothetical social media platform, call it InstaTwitBook, had an algorithm that could accurately judge that a user was suicidal from changes in the language she communicated online. Let's say that site administrators could send this at-risk person a gentle message suggesting that she is showing warning signs of depression, or maybe even nudge her toward

*Pained.* Michael D. Stein and Sandro Galea, Oxford University Press (2020). © Oxford University Press.
DOI: 10.1093/oso/9780197510384.001.0001

help, by sending her advertisements about local mental health counseling. Let's say that 3,500 persons could be reliably identified and sent such messages this year, and that one in 100 messages would lead to care-seeking, averting 35 suicides. Would this not be worthwhile? And it's not just InstaTwitBook that has the power of detection. Phone companies may be able to tell from your voice if you're depressed and use that information to identify who may benefit from mental health help.

Are we comfortable with companies taking such action, if done not in the name of money, but of health? Should InstaTwitBook pursue this public health campaign to save lives, in our era of rising suicide deaths?

It is hard to see why we should not be in favor of this. After all, we accept electronic intrusion for reasons far less consequential than issues of life and death. But there are also challenges that arise from this approach—challenges like inevitable inaccuracy, false-positive results, and the sending of notifications to persons who aren't suicidal. What if there were unintended consequences; what if depressed persons stayed away from social media, growing more isolated, to avoid being singled out?

Answering these questions would take some research; conducting this research would require social media companies to be more open to third-party investigators using their data. Given the reach of social media, and its battered, but still intact, potential for good, such research is long overdue.

## REFERENCES

Chu J. Software listens for hints of depression. *MIT Technology Review*. November 4, 2009. https://www.technologyreview.com/s/416131/software-listens-for-hints-of-depression/ Accessed September 20, 2019.

Eichstaedt JC, Smith RJ, Merchant RM, et al. Facebook language predicts depression in medical records. *Proceedings of the National Academy of Sciences of the United States of America*. 2018; 115(44): 11203–8. doi: 10.1073/pnas.1802331115

Kaste M. Facebook increasingly reliant on A.I. to predict suicide risk. *NPR*. November 17, 2018. https://www.npr.org/2018/11/17/668408122/facebook-increasingly-reliant-on-a-i-to-predict-suicide-risk Accessed September 20, 2019.

Kwon D. Can Facebook's machine-learning algorithms accurately predict suicide? *Scientific American*. March 8, 2017. https://www.scientificamerican.com/article/can-facebooks-machine-learning-algorithms-accurately-predict-suicide/ Accessed September 20, 2019.

Suicide rising across the US. Centers for Disease Control and Prevention Web site. https://www.cdc.gov/vitalsigns/suicide/index.html Accessed September 20, 2019.

Teo AR, Liebow SB, Chan B, Dobscha SK, Graham AL. Reaching those at risk for psychiatric disorders and suicidal ideation: Facebook advertisements to recruit military veterans. *JMIR Mental Health*. 2018; 5(3): e10078. doi: 10.2196/10078

# 55

# RACIAL EQUITY IN KIDNEY TRANSPLANTS

AVERAGE MONTHLY PERCENTAGES
OF WAITLISTED US PATIENTS WHO
RECEIVED A DECEASED-DONOR KIDNEY
TRANSPLANT DURING JUNE 2013–
MARCH 2016, BY RACE/ETHNICITY

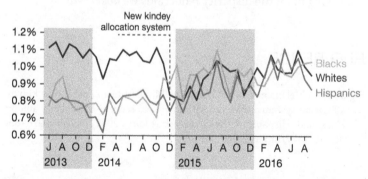

There are stark disparities between the health outcomes of white
people and minorities across a wide range of health indicators.
A prime example is organ transplant allocation. Prior to 2015,
kidney transplants went to white patients at a much higher rate.
A new allocation system was devised in order to change that. The
simple, yet ingenious solution attacked the structural cause of

*Pained*. Michael D. Stein and Sandro Galea, Oxford University Press (2020). © Oxford University Press.
DOI: 10.1093/oso/9780197510384.001.0001

the inequity. It kept time on the donation list as the main selection criteria, but the fix by the United Network for Organ Sharing (UNOS) acknowledged that because of underlying health care disparities, black and Hispanic persons spend more time on dialysis before being put on the list. The new system places the starting point at the earliest date a patient was either put on the list for kidney transplants or started regular dialysis treatments.

Work in *Health Affairs* shows that the new UNOS system worked as intended, and that the racial disparities in transplantation have been largely addressed. Transplants are the go-to treatment option for those with end-stage renal disease, increasing the likelihood of survival and better quality of life, while costing one third as much as long-term dialysis. As the authors of the *Health Affairs* study aptly state: "The new system represents an important step toward achieving equitable access to kidney transplantation, but continued monitoring is crucial to maintaining and improving upon the disparity reductions we observed."

## REFERENCE

Figure from Melanson TA, Hockenberry JM, Plantinga L, et al. New kidney allocation system associated with increased rates of transplants among black and Hispanic patients. *Health Affairs*. 2017; 36(6): 1078–85. doi: 10.1377/hlthaff.2016.1625

# [ 56 ]

# AIR QUALITY STANDARDS
# HAVE ROOM TO IMPROVE

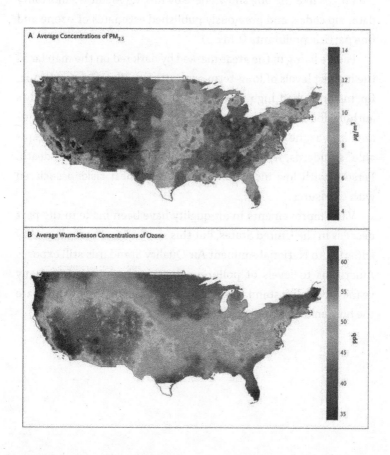

A  Average Concentrations of PM$_{2.5}$

B  Average Warm-Season Concentrations of Ozone

*Pained.* Michael D. Stein and Sandro Galea, Oxford University Press (2020). © Oxford University Press.
DOI: 10.1093/oso/9780197510384.001.0001

The days of US cities with heavy smog so thick you could wipe the grime off your windowsills are, happily, behind us. Laws such as the Clean Air Act (CAA), signed in 1970, resulted in a drastic reduction in air pollution. Emissions have decreased by 50% since then.

Despite these advances, adverse health effects associated with long-term exposure to air pollution continue. Researchers examined the health effects of pollution in a nationwide cohort of 61 million Medicare beneficiaries from 2000 to 2012. They created maps like the one shown here by linking Medicare mortality data, zip codes, and previously published estimates of ozone and fine particle pollutants (PM2.5).

People living in the areas marked by dark red on the map faced the highest levels of long-term exposure to pollutants. California, for instance, had high rates of both pollutants. But the study's authors found that long-term exposures to fine particle pollutants and ozone, even at levels below current nationally "acceptable" standards, were associated with an increased risk of death. Persons with low incomes showed the highest risks associated with exposures.

Vast improvements in air quality have been made in the past decades in the United States, but this study shows that air quality adhering to National Ambient Air Quality Standards still exposes Americans to levels of pollution that can be lethal over many years. Air quality standards must be revisited, in order to alleviate the burden on the most vulnerable populations.

# REFERENCES

Dwyer J. Remembering a city where the smog could kill. *The New York Times.* February 28, 2017. https://www.nytimes.com/2017/02/28/nyregion/ new-york-city-smog.html?_r=0 Accessed September 20, 2019.

Figure from Di Q, Wang Y, Zanobetti A, et al. Air pollution and mortality in the Medicare population. *The New England Journal of Medicine.* 2017; 376(26): 2513–22. doi: 10.1056/NEJMoa1702747. Reproduced with permission.

# WHAT NOBODY WANTS TO TALK ABOUT

*There are certain health topics that we seldom talk about—that we do not want to talk about. We rarely talk about how the justice system is broken and contributes to poor health. That we are supporting an epidemic of alcohol-related death and disability. Or that we have nothing but the most rudimentary approach to the one universal feature of all our lives—our impending death.*

# 57

# BROKEN JUSTICE AND THE PUBLIC'S HEALTH

The incarceration rate in the United States, at 698 per 100,000 people, is higher than any other large country in the world, and nearly five times higher than the median worldwide. There are about 2 million incarcerated adults, or nearly 1 in 100 Americans. Meanwhile, another nearly 5 million people are on probation or parole, for a total of 7 million adults—about 1 in 35 US residents—under correctional supervision.

The chorus of voices showing us how deeply flawed—indeed, broken—our justice system has become is now too loud to ignore. The criminal justice system perpetuates racial inequities that emerge from centuries of disenfranchising minorities in this country. African Americans make up 13% of Americans, but 40% of the incarcerated population. Structural racism, from arrests through the sentencing process, characterizes the criminal justice system. A for-profit bail bond system means that low-level charges can trap lower income families in a cycle of incarceration that can bankrupt them, destroy families, and deepen class divides and attendant health gaps.

Why does this matter to the public's health? First of all, jail and prison are profoundly unhealthy environments. Disability-adjusted life years lost linked to incarceration is over double

*Pained*. Michael D. Stein and Sandro Galea, Oxford University Press (2020). © Oxford University Press.
DOI: 10.1093/oso/9780197510384.001.0001

those attributed to other conditions commonly experienced in the general population. Although prisoners are the only US citizens with a constitutional right to health care, they often face delays in accessing care, restrictive medication formularies, a lack of acute care options, and understaffing of specialty care medical providers, particularly in the areas of mental health and addiction treatment.

But well beyond this, the health effects of our justice system extend into all reaches of the population. A mother's incarceration, for example, is associated with a 30% increase in infant mortality rate, with a stronger effect among blacks than whites. Residents of neighborhoods with high incarceration rates have a two- to threefold increase in rates of depression and anxiety. This likely reflects a combination of the social strain of incarceration among families and a confluence of adverse social circumstances that contributes to increasing incarceration risk in the first place, compounding the challenges faced by communities. There is little question that we consistently underestimate how deeply incarceration influences health.

While a justice system is undoubtedly necessary for social order and safety, a broken justice system compromises the health of the public and deepens the unfairness that characterizes racial health inequities in the country.

## REFERENCES

ACLU National Prison Project. Know your rights: medical, dental and mental health care. American Civil Liberties Union Web site. https://www.aclu. org/files/assets/know_your_rights_--_medical_mental_health_and_ dental_july_2012.pdf Accessed September 20, 2019.

Chen M. Our bail-bond system is broken. *The Nation*. May 11, 2017. https://www.thenation.com/article/our-bail-bond-system-is-broken/ Accessed September 20, 2019.

Daniel AE. Care of the mentally ill in prisons: challenges and solutions. *Journal of the American Academy of Psychiatry and the Law*. 2007; 35(4): 406–10.

Drucker E. *A plague of prisons: the epidemiology of mass incarceration in America*. New York, NY: The New Press; 2011.

Hatzenbuehler ML, Keyes K, Hamilton A, Uddin M, Galea S. The collateral damage of mass incarceration: risk of psychiatric morbidity among non-incarcerated residents of high-incarceration neighborhoods. *American Journal of Public Health*. 2015; 105(1): 138–43.

Walmsley R. World prison population list, eleventh edition. World Prison Brief Web site. https://www.prisonstudies.org/sites/default/files/resources/downloads/world_prison_population_list_11th_edition_0.pdf Accessed September 20, 2019.

Wildeman C. Imprisonment and (inequality in) population health. *Social Science Research*. 2012; 41(1): 74–91.

# 58

# THE PROMISE
# OF PALLIATIVE CARE

As the population ages, patients seeking care for multiple chronic conditions have become the norm. Sixty percent of Americans die following a prolonged illness; a "compression of morbidity"—the limiting of the burden of disease and disability to a brief time before death—has not yet become a reality in the United States. The care of persons with serious chronic illnesses like cancer and heart disease often falls to families, whose members absorb the burden of a loved one's needs, with negative effects on their work, finances, relationships, and community engagement.

Palliative care focuses on improving the quality of life for people with life-threatening illnesses by involving a team of nurses, doctors, social workers, and clergy in a care plan. From its inception nearly 50 years ago, palliative care was meant to provide a system of support for the families of the ill, as well as the patient. Hospice care—administered in dedicated units and in services delivered at home—has been slowly expanded over the past two decades, but the increasing percentage of patients who use hospice for less than 7 days suggests that the full benefits of end-of-life palliative care are not being realized.

Meanwhile, the use of unwanted, aggressive end-of-life care, often inconsistent with patient preferences, remains pervasive.

*Pained.* Michael D. Stein and Sandro Galea, Oxford University Press (2020). © Oxford University Press.
DOI: 10.1093/oso/9780197510384.001.0001

Palliative care programs were designed to help clarify patient wishes, relieve suffering, and improve quality of life throughout an illness, not just at the end of life. Most palliative care is now delivered during hospitalization, when it should be shifting to the community earlier, relieving families from carrying the burden alone.

Community services are currently limited by small numbers of workers and misdirected reimbursement mechanisms; corrective policies have been slow to materialize. And there are other obstacles to progress. The primary one is cultural. When the co-founder of Google announces that he hopes to "cure death," when we believe immortality is achievable through bio-hacking, when the entrepreneurial class chases anti-aging diets, exercise regimens, and technologies, palliative care comes to seem like an admission of failure. Just as Americans have low rates of completing living wills and choosing medical surrogates, they receive few medical referrals to palliative care; doctors notoriously overestimate how long terminally ill patients will live.

Palliative care was not created only for the terminally ill. It can be administered to those who will eventually be cured of an immediate life-threatening condition. It should also engage family caregivers. This public health issue involves not only patients, but also their families, who face material and psychological challenges, and require a comprehensive strategy.

For this strategy to be effective, it must be supported by government policies and insurer incentives; it must also be owned by communities, which must continue to ask for help in designing and paying for high-quality palliative care for patients and their caregiving families.

# REFERENCES

Christakis NA, Lamont EB. Extent and determinants of error in physicians' prognoses in terminally ill patients: prospective cohort study. *Western Journal of Medicine*. 2000; 172(5): 310–13. doi: 10.1136/ewjm.172.5.310

Fries JF. The compression of morbidity. *The Milbank Quarterly*. 2005; 83(4): 801–23. doi: 10.1111/j.1468-0009.2005.00401.x

Teno JM, Gozalo PL, Bynum JP, et al. Change in end-of-life care for Medicare beneficiaries: site of death, place of care, and health care transitions in 2000, 2005, and 2009. *JAMA: The Journal of the American Medical Association*. 2013; 309(5): 470–77. doi: 10.1001/jama.2012.207624.

# REFERENCES

# [ 59 ]

# MAKING AGING HEALTHIER

Today, people are living longer than at any time in human history. The world population of persons aged 65 and older will increase by a factor of 10 between 1950 and 2050, so that, by the middle of the century, there will be about 2.5 times as many adults over age 65 as children under 5.

To address the needs of this aging population we must consider four new realities.

First, healthy aging is the ultimate example of prevention in action. To age in a healthy way, we have to prevent disease from taking hold, suggesting a redoubled effort in preventing some of the conditions—such as obesity and substance use—that result in unhealthy older life.

Second, we must take steps such as creating more accessible built environments, and ensuring older adults have volunteer opportunities, to make sure populations remain integrated in communities as they age.

Third, we must close health gaps that exist among aging populations. These include gaps created by race, LGBTQ status, and socioeconomic status.

And finally, we need to intensify our efforts to tackle the health challenges that older people face. In 2006, there were 26.6 million Alzheimer's disease cases worldwide; that figure is projected to

*Pained.* Michael D. Stein and Sandro Galea, Oxford University Press (2020). © Oxford University Press.
DOI: 10.1093/oso/9780197510384.001.0001

quadruple by 2050, until one in 85 people globally are left with this condition.

While worries about increasing health care costs, coupled with a decline in the wage-earning population, are real, we see increased longevity as the happy result of public health improvements. More important, this demographic shift presents a remarkable moment in human history we would be well advised to recognize and leverage into better health for all.

## REFERENCES

Borji HS. 4 global economic issues of an aging population. Investopedia Web site. https://www.investopedia.com/articles/investing/011216/4-global-economic-issues-aging-population.asp Accessed September 21, 2019.

Brookmeyer R, Johnson E, Ziegler-Graham K, Arrighi HM. Forecasting the global burden of Alzheimer's disease. *Alzheimer's & Dementia: The Journal of the Alzheimer's Association.* 2007; 3(3): 186–91. doi: 10.1016/j.jalz.2007.04.381.

Gurnon E. Why aging and caregiving are harder for LGBT adults. Next Avenue Web site. https://www.nextavenue.org/why-aging-and-caregiving-are-harder-for-lgbt-adults/ Published March 31, 2016. Accessed September 21, 2019.

Healthy places: healthy aging and the built environment. Centers for Disease Control and Prevention Web site. https://www.cdc.gov/healthyplaces/healthtopics/healthyaging.htm Accessed September 21, 2019.

Jaret P. Prices spike for some generic drugs. *AARP Bulletin.* July/August 2015. https://www.aarp.org/health/drugs-supplements/info-2015/prices-spike-for-generic-drugs.html Accessed September 21, 2019.

Research focuses on aging, health among Hispanic women population. Medical News Web site. https://www.news-medical.net/news/20160310/Research-focuses-on-aging-health-among-Hispanic-women-population.aspx Published March 10, 2016. Accessed September 21, 2019.

What are the public health implications of global ageing? World Health Organization Web site. https://www.who.int/features/qa/42/en/ Published September 29, 2011. Accessed September 21, 2019.

# THE DOWNSIDE OF DRINKING

In the midst of a lethal opioid epidemic, alcohol kills more Americans than fentanyl, heroin, and prescription pills combined. During the past decade, in parallel with the increase in opioid use, deaths by alcohol have increased 35%. Although men still make up three quarters of alcohol deaths, young women have had the greatest rise in deaths through accidents, suicide, cancer, and cirrhosis. Alcohol, an ancient substance, seems to have become newly hazardous. Why?

Five potential reasons. First, the alcohol industry continues to be powerful and savvy. Beverage companies spend $2 billion a year on advertising; 90% of this money goes to television ads, mostly for beer. Industry advertising never says that alcohol is not addictive; rather, the message is "use responsibly," which implies that alcohol's use—unlike the use of drugs—is controllable.

Second, although we don't have a greater proportion of Americans drinking (it's remained steady at about two in three people over the past 70 years), we are drinking more, and more easily. We can now buy liquor in movie theaters and in grocery

*Pained.* Michael D. Stein and Sandro Galea, Oxford University Press (2020). © Oxford University Press.
DOI: 10.1093/oso/9780197510384.001.0001

stores and on Sundays. In 2017, Congress reduced alcohol excise taxes, bringing down prices; state legislatures won't raise taxes and risk losing revenue.

Third, during this decade of economic expansion, many Americans have more income. In contrast to the stereotype, affluent people are more likely to drink than low-income people. At the same time, as the poor get poorer, the devastating health effects of heavy drinking are compounded by higher cigarette and other substance use and greater mental health problems.

Fourth, binge-drinking is now a rite of passage in college. With women a growing percentage of collegiate heavy drinkers, and with alcohol-makers targeting women with sweeter and fizzier products, health risks accumulate among women, who generally experience greater alcohol effects at lower doses than men.

Fifth, we've become complacent about driving under the influence, because seatbelts and safer cars have lowered alcohol-related fatalities. Yet, paradoxically, alcohol-related traffic accidents are on the rise (perhaps worsened by growing marijuana co-use). Our drunk-driving blood alcohol threshold remains steady at .08, despite the National Transportation Safety Board's recommendation to lower it to .05, the standard in many other countries with lower rates of traffic fatalities.

We used to think that drinking a little bit had cardio-protective effects. But the science has advanced to show that this is not the case. No level of alcohol consumption improves health. Simply put, alcohol is an eminently preventable cause of social harm and premature death. Consuming less alcohol in total or on a per-occasion basis would probably improve the health of most of us. That's a credible and reasonable public health goal.

# REFERENCES

Alcohol and public health: fact sheets—alcohol use and your health. Centers for Disease Control and Prevention Web site. https://www.cdc.gov/alcohol/fact-sheets/alcohol-use.htm Accessed September 21, 2019.

Burton R, Sheron N. No level of alcohol consumption improves health. *The Lancet*. 2018; 392(10152): 987–988. doi: 10.1016/S0140-6736(18)31571-X

Sareen J, Afifi TO, McMillan KA, Asmundson GJ. Relationship between household income and mental disorders: findings from a population-based longitudinal study. *Archives of General Psychiatry*. 2011; 68(4): 419–427. doi: 10.1001/archgenpsychiatry.2011.15

# [ 61 ]

# HOW FAR DO WOMEN HAVE TO TRAVEL TO GET AN ABORTION?

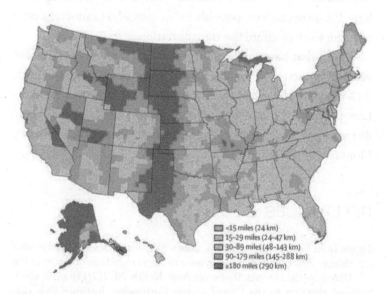

    <15 miles (24 km)
    15–29 miles (24–47 km)
    30–89 miles (48–143 km)
    90–179 miles (145–288 km)
    ≥180 miles (290 km)

Abortion is a common experience for women across the United States. According to the Guttmacher Institute, about one in four women will have an abortion by the age of 45. Access to this care can be affected by a variety of factors, including state laws and policies, socioeconomic status, and geography.

*Pained*. Michael D. Stein and Sandro Galea, Oxford University Press (2020). © Oxford University Press.
DOI: 10.1093/oso/9780197510384.001.0001

As shown in the map, women who want to have an abortion performed in the middle of the country must travel much farther than women living on the coasts to reach a provider. The red areas indicate that women seeking an abortion must travel 180 miles or more. These areas in the middle of the country tend to be rural, while abortion clinics are concentrated in urban settings. Pink areas can also indicate long travel times, ranging from 90 minutes to 3 hours.

The distance needed to travel varies across the country, but it can also vary greatly within a state. In Alaska, about 50% of the women are just over 9 miles away from an abortion provider, but 20% must travel over 150 miles to access care. Traveling these long distances can be impossible for women who cannot take time off from work or afford the transportation costs.

States that have implemented abortion restrictions in recent years have increased the distance women must travel. In Texas, 20% of women have had their travel distance to the nearest abortion provider increase by about 56 miles. Other states where distance and travel times have notably increased include Iowa, Montana, and Missouri.

## REFERENCES

Figure from Bearak JM, Burke KL, Jones RK. Disparities and change over time in distance women would need to travel to have an abortion in the USA: a spatial analysis. *The Lancet Public Health*. 2017; 2(11): e493–e500.

Induced abortion in the United States. Guttmacher Institute Web site. https://www.guttmacher.org/fact-sheet/induced-abortion-united-states#5 Accessed September 21, 2019.

An overview of abortion laws. Guttmacher Institute Web site. https://www.guttmacher.org/state-policy/explore/overview-abortion-laws Accessed September 21, 2019.

Reeves RV, Venator J. Sex, contraception, or abortion? Explaining class gaps in unintended childbearing. Brookings Web site. https://www.brookings. edu/research/sex-contraception-or-abortion-explaining-class-gaps-in-unintended-childbearing/ Published February 26, 2015. Accessed September 21, 2019.

# PLANNING FOR END OF LIFE

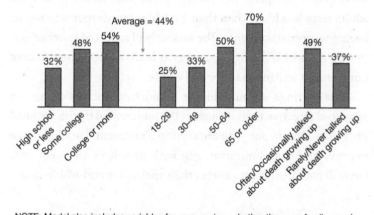

NOTE: Model also includes variables for race, region, whether they or a family member has serious illness, gender, and whether a close friend or a family member has died after a period of serious illness.

SOURCE: kaiser Family Foundation Serious illness in Late Life Survey (conducted May 4-July 12, 2017)

Results of a 2017 survey show that older adults are likelier than younger people to have documented their end-of-life wishes. Yet few adults with or without written documents have discussed end-of-life care with their doctors.

The figure shows that on average, survey respondents had a 44% likelihood of having a written plan or had identified someone to make decisions about their end-of-life care. Age, education, and discussions about death were predictors of having such a plan.

*Pained.* Michael D. Stein and Sandro Galea, Oxford University Press (2020). © Oxford University Press. DOI: 10.1093/oso/9780197510384.001.0001

Those with a college education or higher were most likely to have a written document, compared to those with some college, high school, or less education. Also, talking about death while growing up correlated with having written documents about wishes for medical care.

As expected, adults aged 65 or older were most likely to have a written document or to name someone to take charge of their medical decisions. Although older adults were likelier to have some end-of-life plan, the survey found that seriously ill older adults were less likely than their healthier counterparts to report having written documents. The seriously ill reported lower education levels, which the figure depicts as being a strong predictor of not having a written plan for end-of-life.

Care settings encouraging or mandating doctors to use an advanced directive toolkit, such as the one created by the National Physician Orders for Life-Sustaining Treatment Paradigm, can improve the communication gap with providers and help seriously ill patients better express their wishes for end-of-life care.

## REFERENCES

Figure from DiJulio B, Hamel L, Wu B, Brodie M. Serious illness in late life: The public's views and experiences. Kaiser Family Foundation Web site. https://www.kff.org/report-section/serious-illness-in-late-life-the-publics-views-and-experiences-section-3-documenting-and-talking-about-wishes/. Published November 2, 2017. Accessed September 21, 2019.

Goldberg L. New toolkit bolsters end-of-life resources. The Pew Charitable Trusts Web site. https://www.pewtrusts.org/en/research-and-analysis/articles/2018/02/02/new-toolkit-bolsters-end-of-life-resources. Published February 2, 2018. Accessed September 21, 2019.

# SECTION 10

# MAKING THINGS BETTER

*How can the engaged citizen take matters in her own hands, to improve the health of the public? How can we leverage existing institutions and community networks into better health for all?*

# [ 63 ]

# VOLUNTEERING FOR THE HEALTH OF THE PUBLIC

The world is aging rapidly. There are now more people over the age of 65 than under the age of 5 worldwide. And we all want to age in a healthy way.

Of the many ways to facilitate healthy aging, one is especially simple and available to all: volunteering. There is a strong link between volunteering and good health. Formal volunteering (outside the home, for the good of others) has been associated with reduced mortality and increased self-rated health and physical function. Indeed, 2018 research suggests that those who have the greatest health vulnerabilities are, in fact, most likely to experience positive health benefits from volunteering.

How does volunteering help? It can increase physical activity, social engagement, and brain stimulation. It may decrease social isolation, as new friendships emerge from the shared experience of volunteering. It can promote confidence and enhance one's sense of meaning and purpose. Volunteering might be particularly beneficial to cognitive functioning because it allows older adults to engage in, and master, complex tasks, many of which might be new to them.

How many weekly volunteer hours are necessary to produce these positive results? The evidence suggests relatively few,

*Pained*. Michael D. Stein and Sandro Galea, Oxford University Press (2020). © Oxford University Press.
DOI: 10.1093/oso/9780197510384.001.0001 .

although there may be a dose effect. Maintenance is key, and it is probably easiest via forms of volunteering that are relevant to one's life and experience.

One of the greatest challenges in this era of rapid population aging is to develop public health interventions that effectively decrease the number of years older people spend disabled. The potential for volunteer engagement as an innovative and significant public health disability reduction intervention should get our attention. The cherry on top is that estimates already place the value of volunteer service at nearly $200 billion per year.

This seems like an extraordinary opportunity. If we can encourage more volunteering in the growing elderly population, we can create a social good that also improves the health of the volunteer. As a society, we should invest in making volunteering a routine part of growing older, a way to create a world where aging is full of opportunities for good health.

## REFERENCES

Carr DC, Kail BL, Rowe JW. The relation of volunteering and subsequent changes in physical disability in older adults. *The Journals of Gerontology: Series B.* 2017; 73(3): 511–21. doi: 10.1093/geronb/gbx102

New report: service unites Americans; volunteers give service worth $184 billion. Corporation for National and Community Service Web site. https://www.nationalservice.gov/newsroom/press-releases/2016/new-report-service-unites-americans-volunteers-give-service-worth-184 Published November 15, 2016. Accessed September 21, 2019.

Proulx CM, Curl AL, Ermer AE. Longitudinal associations between formal volunteering and cognitive functioning. *The Journals of Gerontology: Series B.* 2017; 73(3): 522–31. doi: 10.1093/geronb/gbx110.

# 64

# MENTAL HEALTH ON CAMPUS

College students experience many highs and lows. But, sadly, the lows appear to have deepened. More than 10% of today's students report suicidal thoughts, the highest rate since widespread campus surveying began. College counselors point to growing stress among students, with more than a third reporting that they have been diagnosed with a mental health condition, most often anxiety or depression, but also, increasingly, with eating disorders and forms of self-harm. There is considerable variation across schools, not explained by school size or competitiveness, but there remains a consistently higher prevalence of all mental health problems among students from lower socioeconomic backgrounds (financial stress is the most common risk factor) and among students with minority gender and sexual orientations.

While only a small proportion of students report they would think less of someone who has received mental health treatment, few avail themselves of such services. Only about half of students with apparent symptoms seek formal care. Many prefer to deal with issues on their own or believe that they don't have enough time to get help. Others question the seriousness of their needs, believing that overwhelming stress is normal in college, or that problems will get better on their own. Stigma remains on campuses insofar as students don't think their fellow students share

*Pained.* Michael D. Stein and Sandro Galea, Oxford University Press (2020). © Oxford University Press.
DOI: 10.1093/oso/9780197510384.001.0001

attitudes as generous as their own toward those with mental health problems.

There is a clear-cut case for investment in campus mental health services: 30% of depressed students eventually drop out, and research suggests that one fifth of this drop-out rate can be averted by early intervention and treatment. This means that for every 500 incoming students, a robust mental health system would help 30 more complete college, adding about $1 million in tuition to that school. Based on the cost of providing mental health services, for every $1 spent on such services, there is a $2 increase in school revenue.

This calculation presents only a narrow perspective. Since life-time earnings follow from successful graduation, there is even greater value to an at-risk student if he or she is not derailed by a mental health problem during college. Screening and intervention programs are investments in academic achievement, and they will have downstream effects on the public's health.

Untreated mental health problems are connected to every aspect of student life. The eating, sleeping, and drinking behaviors of college students continue to be maladaptive, leading to increased ill effects. Mental health service providers at and around campuses are busy. They should probably be busier.

## REFERENCES

Bradley BJ, Greene AC. Do health and education agencies in the United States share responsibility for academic achievement and health? A review of 25 years of evidence about the relationship of adolescents' academic achievement and health behaviors. *Journal of Adolescent Health*. 2013; 52(5): 523–32. doi: 10.1016/j.jadohealth.2013.01.008

Eisenberg D, Hunt J, Speer N. Mental health in American colleges and universities: variation across student subgroups and across campuses. *The*

*Journal of Nervous and Mental Disease.* 2013; 201(1): 60–67. doi: 10.1097/NMD.0b013e31827ab077

Gaddis SM, Ramirez D, Hernandez EL. Contextualizing public stigma: Endorsed mental health treatment stigma on college and university campuses. *Social Science & Medicine.* 2018; 197:183–91. doi: 10.1016/j.socscimed.2017.11.029

# 65

# HEALTHY HOMES

Sixteen million American children live in poverty, putting them at risk for delayed development, disease, and poor educational outcomes. The Earned Income Tax Credit (EITC) is a pro-work, federal tool that has reduced or eliminated poverty for 13.2 million children. Cash transfer programs like EITC improve maternal and infant health.

But 20% of eligible households do not claim this tax credit. More problematically, families who do seek the refund give away 15%–20% of it ($1.75 billion yearly) to for-profit tax preparers.

To lower the US poverty rate, which has plateaued, how might health systems help families maximize this economic credit?

Pediatricians are uniquely positioned, trusted professionals, who interact regularly with low-income families; over 90% of children under 2 years old see a doctor yearly. A 2018 program suggests it is possible to connect EITC-eligible families to free tax preparation through physician referral, fliers included with visit reminders, in-clinic advertising, and calls to families with upcoming appointments in the pediatric clinic, offering tax services 15 to 25 hours weekly, including evenings and weekends. Walk-in visits to a tax preparer, in conjunction with a medical appointment, are available. Families arrive 15 minutes early to complete intake, go to their appointment while taxes are prepared by

*Pained.* Michael D. Stein and Sandro Galea, Oxford University Press (2020). © Oxford University Press.
DOI: 10.1093/oso/9780197510384.001.0001

trained volunteer professionals, and return to finalize their return after the physician visit. Grants, corporate donations, and private philanthropy are used to cover central programming costs (one full-time staff salary, marketing materials, computers).

The program was associated with increased filing rates, receipt of EITC (average $605 refund), and use of free tax preparation, all of which increase money for low-income families. Participants felt more connected to their doctor than persons who didn't join the program.

Finding such clever, convenient ways to make better use of federal policies to reduce poverty one family at a time creates a novel community resource. Doctors' offices are one of the only places all families with young children frequent. Targeting predominantly minority, low-income, and Medicaid-insured patients, many of whom are non-English speaking, such on-site, tax returns programs, if disseminated, will permit families to share their financial struggles and enhance the EITC's underestimated pro-work effect.

For all the talk of the patient-centered "medical home"—a team-based approach for better health outcomes—programs like this one, with a wider view of health creation, are the beginning of a new model: "healthy homes."

## REFERENCES

Hoynes HW, Patel AJ. Effective policy for reducing inequality? The Earned Income Tax Credit and the distribution of income. The National Bureau of Economic Research Web site. https://www.nber.org/papers/w21340 Accessed September 22, 2019.

Marcil LE, Hole MK, Wenren LM, Schuler MS, Zuckerman BS, Vinci RJ. Free tax services in pediatric clinics. *Pediatrics*. 2018; 141(6).

Tax Policy Center briefing book: key elements of the US tax system. Tax Policy Center Web site. https://www.taxpolicycenter.org/briefing-book/what-earned-income-tax-credit Accessed September 22, 2019.

Weinstein Jr P, Patten B. The price of paying taxes II: How paid tax preparer fees are diminishing the Earned Income Tax Credit (EITC). Progressive Policy Institute Web site. https://www.progressivepolicy.org/wp-content/uploads/2016/04/2016.04-Weinstein_Patten_The-Price-of-Paying-Takes-II.pdf Accessed September 22, 2019.

# 66

# TOWARD A MUSCULAR PUBLIC HEALTH

Public health often offers directives. You should wear seat belts. You should get vaccinated. You shouldn't smoke. This command language, with its moral tinge, is at odds with the language of shared decision-making that has become central to the medical world, and which, in some ways, may marginalize the message of public health.

Why does public health embrace an approach that can seem at odds both with notions of individual freedom and medical norms? In the shared decision-making world of modern medicine, doctors are meant to discuss options with patients, with the final health decision made by the patient, who may, in the end, make an unhealthy choice. But public health persists in suggesting courses of actions for the entire population, to be taken on a population's behalf.

## WHY?

The answer is simple. Public health professionals know best for populations; individuals know best for themselves.

*Pained*. Michael D. Stein and Sandro Galea, Oxford University Press (2020). © Oxford University Press.
DOI: 10.1093/oso/9780197510384.001.0001

Let's use smoking cigarettes as an example. Public health professionals are delighted that the prevalence of smoking has decreased from 50% to 16% in the past five decades. A future elimination of all tobacco use would be even better—the end of smoking would save millions more lives. Smoking's end, when it comes, will be caused by the same factors that drove smoking's decline—decisions made by public health professionals to improve the health of populations.

Shared decision-making is necessary at medical visits; clinical providers may be experts, but the best data about treatment may not apply to the patient in the office, and so outcomes are always in doubt. Hence, the patient can reasonably choose for herself among a number of uncertain options. But we can be much more certain about outcomes when we are considering the health of populations. By any reasonable measure—longevity, cost to the health system, quality of life—smokers do worse than nonsmokers. We can say this with certainty. After assembling incontrovertible evidence—in this case, of the hazards of smoking—public health providers try to universalize its application for the good of all. So we tax cigarettes, we institute anti-smoking advertising campaigns, and we increase insurance premiums to smokers, all to create a healthier population.

Society entrusts public health to understand what is in the public good and to act on it. Therefore, when we know the healthiest answer, we should be relentless in seeking its implementation. It is up to society to decide if public health should or should not be in a position to flex its muscles. But, when we see opportunity to improve the public's health, which derives from the combination of evidence and public agreement, we should act, even in the absence of consensus.

# 67

# ZERO TOLERANCE FOR PREVENTABLE DEATHS

Of the approximately 150,000 daily deaths around the world, about a third are preventable (the rest are age-related, hence non-preventable). In the United States, more than 400,000 people die annually due to smoking, and more than 300,000 due to poor diet—these are the leading causes of preventable deaths.

The good news is that the number of preventable deaths is declining in the United States. Preventable deaths from cancer, injuries, stroke, and heart disease decreased by 25%, 23%, 11%, and 4%, respectively, in the first 5 years of the 2010s. And we can reduce the number of preventable deaths further. An analysis conducted by the CDC found that if we were to reduce the number of preventable deaths across all states to the levels found in the three states with the lowest preventable death rates, we would prevent 91,891 deaths from heart diseases, 84,539 from cancer, 37,016 from unintentional injuries, 28,853 from chronic lower respiratory diseases, and 17,062 from stroke, for a total of more than 250,000 deaths prevented annually, or nearly 10% of annual deaths in the United States.

Should it not occasion headlines that we can prevent more than a quarter million deaths a year but choose not to? Maybe the reason we do not see such headlines is because they might motivate

*Pained.* Michael D. Stein and Sandro Galea, Oxford University Press (2020). © Oxford University Press.
DOI: 10.1093/oso/9780197510384.001.0001

us to take on the difficult task of preventing these deaths. This would require a tremendous effort to lessen risk behaviors and deal with the foundational social, economic, and environmental forces that shape health. The hard, slow work this would entail is perhaps why we have mostly avoided it, only spending a mere 5% of our health dollars on prevention.

But let us entertain a thought exercise. There are 4 billion airline passengers a year worldwide. What if there were 10,000 deaths annually from air crashes? We would call these preventable—after all, most people who fly do not expect to die. And what if we knew that we could reduce these deaths if all airlines behaved like the three safest ones? Would we then refuse to take action? Of course not. We would find this situation intolerable, because we have zero tolerance for any deaths from flying—we find each death unacceptable. It is remarkable that we have figured out how to fly 4 billion people around the world annually with minimal deaths. It is equally remarkable that we are not focused on the early interventions, risk factor reduction programs, and public health efforts that can dramatically reduce preventable deaths.

## REFERENCES

CDC estimates preventable deaths from 5 leading causes. Centers for Disease Control and Prevention Web site. https://www.cdc.gov/media/releases/2016/p1117-preventable-deaths.html Accessed September 22, 2019.

Hermosilla SC, Kujawski SA, Richards CA, Muennig PA, Galea S, El-Sayed AM. An ounce of prevention: deaths averted from primary prevention interventions. *American Journal of Preventive Medicine.* 2017; 52(6): 778–87. doi: 10.1016/j.amepre.2017.01.002

Percentage of deaths in the U.S. that were potentially preventable in 2015, by cause. Statista Web site. https://www.statista.com/statistics/791565/

percentage-of-preventable-deaths-united-states-by-cause/  Accessed September 22, 2019.

Yoon PW, Bastian B, Anderson RN, Collins JL, Jaffe HW. Potentially preventable deaths from the five leading causes of death—United States, 2008–2010. *Morbidity and Mortality Weekly Report (MMWR).* 2014; 63(17): 369–74.

# [ 68 ]

# POLICE AND THE
# PUBLIC'S HEALTH

Police work is community work. Performed on the street, in public settings and private homes, police work shapes the health context of cities and neighborhoods, and affects the lives and behaviors of countless citizens. While there has been much concern in recent years—appropriately—about how some police activity has harmed health, particularly among minority communities, police have the potential to improve the health of the communities they serve.

Most police interaction with the public does not involve major crimes or violence, or require arrest or use of force. Police beat work is filled with low-intensity interactions in which officers serve as problem-solvers; these problems often involve public health.

Police regularly find themselves at the center of our national public health crises. They are first responders to opioid overdoses; they intercede in intimate partner violence, and they engage with the homeless. Leveraging police involvement into better health outcomes could go a long way toward helping us solve these crises.

For a template for how we could do this, we need look no further than how police interact with the mentally ill. One in 10 police contacts with the public in the United States involves

*Pained.* Michael D. Stein and Sandro Galea, Oxford University Press (2020). © Oxford University Press.
DOI: 10.1093/oso/9780197510384.001.0001

persons with serious mental illnesses. Police officers are trained in self-defense and often think in terms of force and arrest. Yet officers now commonly transport people to hospital emergency departments for psychiatric evaluation rather than to jail. In the field, officers must be creative and persuasive to avoid unnecessary arrests.

Increasingly, large cities are developing crisis intervention teams (CITs) to improve safety and divert individuals from criminal justice involvement. CIT training involves learning the signs and symptoms of mental illness and the threats it can pose, and allowing officers to spend time with mentally ill persons, their families, and mental health service providers, as well as learning new negotiation tactics and decision-making skills.

In places where CIT takes hold, police officers do preventive work—they engage with families and manage complex mental health needs. In this way, police serve as front-line public health workers, linking individuals to treatment and other resources that can inflect the trajectory of a person's life for the good.

CIT training is currently voluntary (and selective) in a limited number of police forces. Implemented more widely, such training can support a cultural shift toward improved de-escalation and diversion practices in law enforcement. Such an investment of police time and resources, if broadened to cover other areas of public health consequence, could have a powerful, positive effect on the health of communities.

## REFERENCES

Black Lives Matter Web site. https://blacklivesmatter.com/ Accessed September 22, 2019.

Bor J, Venkataramani AS, Williams DR, Tsai AC. Police killings and their spillover effects on the mental health of black Americans: a population-based, quasi-experimental study. *The Lancet.* 2018; 392(10144): 302–10. doi: 10.1016/S0140-6736(18)31130-9

The Police Assisted Addiction and Recovery Initiative Web site. https://paari-usa.org/ Accessed September 22, 2019.

President's Task Force on 21st Century Policing. *Final report of the President's Task Force on 21st Century Policing.* Washington, DC: Office of Community Oriented Policing Services; 2015.

Schiff DM, Drainoni ML, Weinstein ZM, Chan L, Bair-Merritt M, Rosenbloom D. A police-led addiction treatment referral program in Gloucester, MA: implementation and participants' experiences. *Journal of Substance Abuse Treatment.* 2017; 82: 41–47. doi: 10.1016/j.jsat.2017.09.003

Watson AC, Ottati VC, Morabito M, Draine J, Kerr AN, Angell B. Outcomes of police contacts with persons with mental illness: the impact of CIT. *Administration and Policy in Mental Health and Mental Health Services Research.* 2010; 37(4): 302–17. doi: 10.1007/s10488-009-0236-9

# 69

# MAKING STRIDES
# TOWARD ZERO

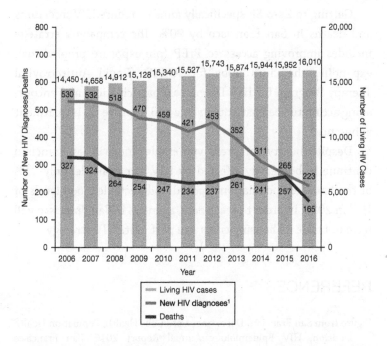

San Francisco has made steady progress toward fulfilling its goals of achieving zero HIV deaths, zero new infections, and zero HIV stigma by 2020. These goals are aligned with the UNAIDS Fast-Track strategy for reaching the three zeros globally.

*Pained.* Michael D. Stein and Sandro Galea, Oxford University Press (2020). © Oxford University Press.
DOI: 10.1093/oso/9780197510384.001.0001

In its annual report for 2016, the San Francisco Department of Public Health's HIV Epidemiology section summed up data on new and existing HIV infections and HIV-related deaths in the city. As shown in the figure, the number of new HIV diagnoses decreased steadily between 2007 and 2012, when there was a brief uptick in new cases. By 2013, incidence resumed its downward trajectory. The number of people living with HIV went up each year due to life-saving treatment. HIV-related deaths held fairly steady between 2008 and 2015, before dropping dramatically in 2016.

Getting to Zero SF specifically aims to reduce HIV infections and deaths in San Francisco by 90%. The campaign's strategy includes improving access to PrEP (pre-exposure prophylaxis), expanding the city's hubs for RAPID (Rapid Antiretroviral Therapy Program for HIV Diagnoses) participation, and encouraging action to keep patients in care and improve their treatment adherence.

Despite the city's progress, vulnerable groups in San Francisco continue to be heavily affected by HIV. For example, only 31% of the homeless population reached undetectable blood levels of HIV in 2016. In order to reach zero, agencies in San Francisco will have to tackle its housing crisis as a part of its HIV strategy.

## REFERENCES

Figure from San Francisco Department of Public Health, Population Health Division. HIV Epidemiology Annual Report 2016. San Francisco Department of Public Health Web site. https://www.sfdph.org/dph/files/reports/RptsHIVAIDS/Annual-Report-2016-20170831.pdf. Accessed September 22, 2019.

Getting to Zero SF Web site. http://www.gettingtozerosf.org. Accessed September 22, 2019.

Highleyman L. San Francisco annual report shows continued drop in new HIV infections. aidsmap Web site. http://www.aidsmap.com/news/sep-2017/san-francisco-annual-report-shows-continued-drop-new-hiv-infections. Accessed September 22, 2019.

UNAIDS Strategy 2016–2021. Joint United Nations Programme on HIV/AIDS Web site. https://www.unaids.org/en/resources/documents/2015/UNAIDS_PCB37_15-18 Accessed September 22, 2019.

# 70

# CANCER SURVIVAL IS (MOSTLY) IMPROVING

Five-year cancer survival rates in the USA
Average five-year survival rates from common cancer types in the United States,
shown as the rate over the period 1970–77 [•] and over the period 2007–2013 [•]: 1970–77 •———• 2007–2013
This five-year interval indicates the perventage of people who live longer than five years following diagnosis.

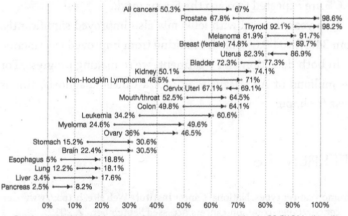

Based on data by Journal of the National Cancer Institute;
Surveillance, Epidemiology and End Results Program.
The data visualization is available at OurWorldinData.org.
There you find research and more visualizations on this topic.

Licensed under CC-BY-SA by the authors
Hannah Ritchie and Max Roser.

The 5-year survival rates for the most common cancers in the United States improved by nearly 20% (see first line of the graph) since the 1970s. While promising overall, low survival rates persist for pancreatic, liver, lung, esophageal, brain, and many other

*Pained.* Michael D. Stein and Sandro Galea, Oxford University Press (2020). © Oxford University Press.
DOI: 10.1093/oso/9780197510384.001.0001

cancers. Five-year survival for uterine and cervical cancers worsened, and researchers aren't sure why.

Lung cancer remains the most common type of cancer across the globe, with nearly 2.1 million diagnoses worldwide. In the United States, approximately 234,000 Americans were diagnosed in 2018. Despite its extremely high prevalence, only 18.1% of individuals with a lung cancer diagnosis (up from 12.2%) are expected to reach their 5-year survival mark.

Pancreatic cancer has the lowest 5-year survival rate at 8.2%.

In contrast, prostate cancer had the greatest 5-year survival increase from 67.8% to 98.6%, most likely reflecting a substantial uptick in prostate cancer screening and early detection. Of the 165,000 Americans diagnosed with prostate cancer in 2018, 98.6% are expected to reach the 5-year mark.

Five-year survival with leukemia also improved significantly, from 34.2% to 60.6%, likely resulting from improved treatments.

In both detection and treatment, we're making progress. For the millions of Americans who face a cancer diagnosis, this is cause for hope.

## REFERENCES

Common cancer types. National Cancer Institute Web site. https://www.cancer.gov/types/common-cancers Accessed September 22, 2019.

Figure from Roser M, Ritchie H. Cancer. Our World in Data Web site. https://ourworldindata.org/cancer#cancer-survival-rates Accessed September 22, 2019.

Lung cancer fact sheet. American Lung Association Web site. https://www.lung.org/lung-health-and-diseases/lung-disease-lookup/lung-cancer/resource-library/lung-cancer-fact-sheet.html Accessed September 22, 2019.

# INDEX

*For the benefit of digital users, indexed terms that span two pages (e.g., 52–53) may, on occasion, appear on only one of those pages.*